AF556816

Descent of the Testis

To Susan, Lin,
Kathleen, Andrew,
John, Sarah,
Rowena, Matthew,
Julia and Iain.

Descent of the Testis

John M. Hutson,
MB BS (Monash), MD(Melb), FRACS

Senior Lecturer in Paediatric Surgery,
Department of Paediatrics, University of Melbourne
and Deputy Chairman, Department of General Surgery,
Royal Children's Hospital, Melbourne

and

Spencer W. Beasley,
MB ChB(Otago), MS(Melb), FRACS

Senior Lecturer in Paediatric Surgery (Part-time),
Department of Paediatrics, University of Melbourne
and Consultant Paediatric Surgeon, Royal Children's Hospital,
Melbourne, and Preston & Northcote Community Hospital,
Melbourne

Edward Arnold
A division of Hodder & Stoughton
LONDON MELBOURNE AUCKLAND

First published in Great Britain 1992

British Library Cataloguing in Publication Data

Hutson, John M.
Descent of the Testis
I. Title II. Beasley, Spencer W.
618.92

ISBN 0–340–55400–2

Whilst the advice and information in this book is believed to be true and accurate at the date of going to press, neither the author nor the publisher can accept any legal responsibility or liability for any errors or omissions that may be made. In particular (but without limiting the generality of the preceding disclaimer) every effort has been made to check drug dosages; however, it is still possible that errors have been missed. Furthermore, dosage schedules are constantly being revised and new side effects recognised. For these reasons the reader is strongly urged to consult the drug companies' printed instructions before administering any of the drugs recommended in this book.

Typeset in 10/12pt Palatino by Anneset, Weston-super-Mare, Avon. Printed and bound in Great Britain for Edward Arnold, a division of Hodder and Stoughton Limited, Mill Road, Dunton Green, Sevenoaks, Kent TN13 2YA by Butler & Tanner Ltd, Frome and London.

Contents

Acknowledgements

This book would not have been possible without the dedicated assistance of Mrs Elizabeth Vorrath, Mrs Judith Hayes, Mrs Veronica Bello and Miss Kathleen Hutson. Many colleagues contributed photos or artwork and their assistance is greatly appreciated and acknowledged in the figure legends. The publishing companies are thanked for kindly giving permission to reproduce numerous figures. Finally, the authors thank Mr Paul Price of Edward Arnold for encouraging us to produce this monograph.

Introduction

Descent of the testis, or lack thereof, is a subject of great controversy in embryology, endocrinology and paediatric surgery. For such a common abnormality as undescended testis, it is surprising that there remain so many unanswered questions:

(1) Why does the testis descend?
(2) How does the testis descend?
(3) What causes undescended testes?
(4) What is the best treatment for maldescent?
(5) Does hormone therapy have a role in treatment and/or diagnosis?
(6) Are there any new alternatives to surgical treatment?
(7) When is the optimal time for treatment?
(8) Are 'retractile' testes normal or abnormal?
(9) Do retractile/ascending testes need treatment?
(10) What is the cause of infertility and increased malignancy?
(11) Will fertility improve and the risk of cancer diminish with current modes of treatment?
(12) Will early surgery prevent testicular degeneration?

This book aims to present up-to-date evidence from our own and other laboratories of the normal mechanisms of testicular descent (Chapters 2–3), along with a brief description of the evolution of descent and the early history of research of its cause (Chapter 1).

Chapters 4–9 describe the clinical problems of undescended testes and give our own, necessarily biased, opinions of the best ways to diagnose and treat the anomaly. We have not emphasized hormonal treatment, which has been vigorously proposed by others in recent years, for two major reasons. First, current evidence now suggests that direct or indirect stimulation of androgen secretion only causes relaxation of the cremaster muscle in 'retractile' testes, but has little effect on truly undescended testes. Secondly, luteinizing hormone-releasing hormone (LHRH) or its long-acting analogues, have not been approved for clinical use in Australia, and therefore we have no direct experience of their use. Human chorionic gonadotrophin (hCG) is available, but its not in general use because of lack of efficacy and the need for a significant number of painful injections.

The descriptions of the clinical diagnosis (Chapter 6) and the surgical treatment (Chapter 7) are given in detail, with extensive pictorial support, so as to give the trainee surgeon enough information to be able to learn exactly what we do. We have opted for a detailed description of orchidopexy as it is performed currently by us and our colleagues at the Royal Children's Hospital, Melbourne. Previous surgical techniques, such as the Torek fixation of the testis to the thigh with rubber bands (!), have been omitted deliberately because they were cruel, unnecessary, or caused testicular atrophy. There is now no place for such methods in modern paediatric surgery, where the goal is to perform day-case surgery with minimal pain or discomfort to the hapless infant or child. With this approach, orchidopexy can be performed without any painful injections or unpleasant memories.

The long-term results of current surgical treatment (Chapter 9) remain unknown, but we are optimistic that surgery in infancy will lead to a significant improvement in fertility and reduced risk of malignancy.

Chapter 10 concludes this short monograph with an attempt to summarize our answers to the list of questions given above. Inevitably, some of our answers will be found wanting in the future, but they will serve as a guide to future advances. Finally, we speculate on the ways that undescended testes may be treated in the future, based on our research into normal mechanisms of descent and the physiology of the testis.

There are many areas of the subject that we have not dealt with extensively; the reader should consult those books that address these areas directly. For a classic description of the human problems, the reader could do no better than read Scorer and Farrington's 1971 treatise[1]: we have attempted unashamedly to emulate its style and approach. During the 1970s and early 1980s, the dominant paradigm was the central role of the hypothalamic–pituitary–gonadal axis which provided the rationale for hormone treatment. Several good multi-authored volumes appeared at that time, with extensive discussion of all endocrine aspects of the problem.[2–4] A more up-to-date discussion of endocrine effects appeared in the *European Journal of Paediatrics* on the occasion of the 125th Anniversary of the Children's Hospital, Basle.[5] The role of hormones in treatment was questioned in 1986 by de Muinck Keizer-Schrama and Hazebroek in their joint thesis from Erasmus University, Rotterdam.[6] Two recent reviews include Abney and Keel's[7] volume that contains detailed articles on the effect of maldescent on the endocrine system, and Schier and Waldschmidt's[8] edited proceedings of a combined medical and surgical meeting in Berlin in 1988.

References

1. Scorer CG, Farrington GH. *Congenital Deformities of the Testis and Epididymis*. London: Butterworths, 1971.
2. Bierich JR, Giarola A. *Cryptorchidism, Proceedings of the Serono Symposia*. London: Academic Press, 1979, Vol. 25.
3. Fonkalsrud EW, Mengel W. *The Undescended Testis*. Chicago: Year Book Medical Publishers, 1981.
4. Hadziselimovic F (ed). *Cryptorchidism, Management and Implications*. Berlin: Springer-Verlag, 1983.
5. Hadziselimovic F, Herzog B, Girard J (eds). *Eur J Pediatr* 1987; **146** (Suppl 2): S1–S68.
6. De Muinck Keizer-Schrama SMPF, Hazebroek FWJ. *The Treatment of Cryptorchidism. Why, How, When?* Theses, Erasmus University, Rotterdam, 1986.
7. Abney TO, Keel BA (eds). *The Cryptorchid Testis*. Boca Raton, Florida: CRC Press, 1989.
8. Schier F, Waldschmidt J (eds). *Padiatrie aktuell 1: Maldescensus testis*. Munchen: W Zukerschwerdt Verlag, 1990.

1

Evolution of descent of the testis and early history of research

1.1 Evolution of testicular descent

1.1.1 Why is the testis descended at all?

Early vertebrates had intra-abdominal gonads, regardless of sex. With subsequent evolution of sexual differences the testis has acquired a different position from the ovary, presumably because this different position has conferred some biological advantage. It is not known exactly why evolution has produced descended testes outside the abdominal cavity, although the scrotum has undoubtedly become a highly specialized low-temperature environment. Bedford[1] proposed that descent of the testis is merely a secondary phenomenon accompanying descent of the epididymis. Since early vertebrates, such as fish, probably ejaculated the semen into the environment, spermatozoa could have acquired advantage by being adapted to environmental temperatures below that of the body: the storage organ for spermatozoa also might benefit from adaptations to cooler temperatures. In animals where the testis is not normally descended into a pendulous scrotum, the caudal epididymis where sperm are stored is the most superficial genital organ, and hence is maintained at a lower temperature than the internal organs. The testis as the site of production of spermatozoa also may have acquired evolutionary advantage, being at a lower temperature.

Most mammals have acquired a large number of sophisticated anatomical and physiological adaptations of the scrotum to keep the epididymis and testis cool (Table 1.1), many of which are present in the human. Because the human testis has inherited major adaptations fitting it to exist at a lower temperature than the body core, any disruption of normal descent would be expected to upset testicular physiology, as is discussed in Chapter 5.

Table 1.1 The scrotum as a low-temperature environment

Character	Physiological role
Thin, pigmented skin	Heat loss by conduction/radiation
No subcutaneous fat	Heat loss by conduction
Absent hair/fur (e.g. rat)	Heat loss over caudal epididymis
Pampiform plexus	Counter-current heat exchange
Cremaster muscle	Controls dependency of testis in response to external temperatures
Dartos muscle	Controls scrotal dependency in response to external temperature
Fat pad in inguinal canal (e.g. rat)	Insulates testis from abdominal cavity
Fat pad between testis and epididymis (rat)	Insulates caudal epididymis from testis
Processus vaginalis obliteration	Keeps testis outside abdominal wall

The different anatomical and physiological characteristics found in different species are important for an overall understanding of human testicular descent because they reveal the various phases through which the mechanism has passed. Some of these phases may be concealed by idiosyncratic anatomical features, but the basic mechanism of testicular descent should be present in increasing complexity.

1.1.2 Which animals have descended testes?

Descent of the testis from its initial position on the urogenital ridge to the scrotum occurs only in mammals. Other vertebrates, such as fish and birds (Figure 1.1), have testes which remain inside the abdomen. Monotremes, such as the platypus and the spiny ant-eater or echidna (Figure 1.2), form an intermediate group between mammals and other vertebrates and have high, intra-abdominal testes.[2] By contrast with the platypus and echidna, marsupials such as the kangaroo exhibit complete testicular descent (Figure 1.3)[3,4]

Some eutherian mammals have intra-abdominal testes which remain in their original position on the urogenital ridge. These include such widely different animals as the elephant and the rock hyrax (a small African herbivore) (Figure 1.4).[5,6] The elephant (Figure 1.5) and the hyrax appear to have no structure analogous to the gubernaculum. Aquatic mammals (porpoises, dolphins and whales) have testes which are partially descended within the abdomen (Figure 1.6a,b).[7,8] Meek has speculated that aquatic mammals had descended testes during an earlier epoch, but this feature has been lost to a variable extent in subsequent millenia.

In the narwhale (Figure 1.6c)[8] and the prairie dog (Figure 1.7),[9] the testes are lateral to the bladder neck and are just inside the inguinal region. Hedgehogs, moles and shrews have testes lying lateral to the bladder; in

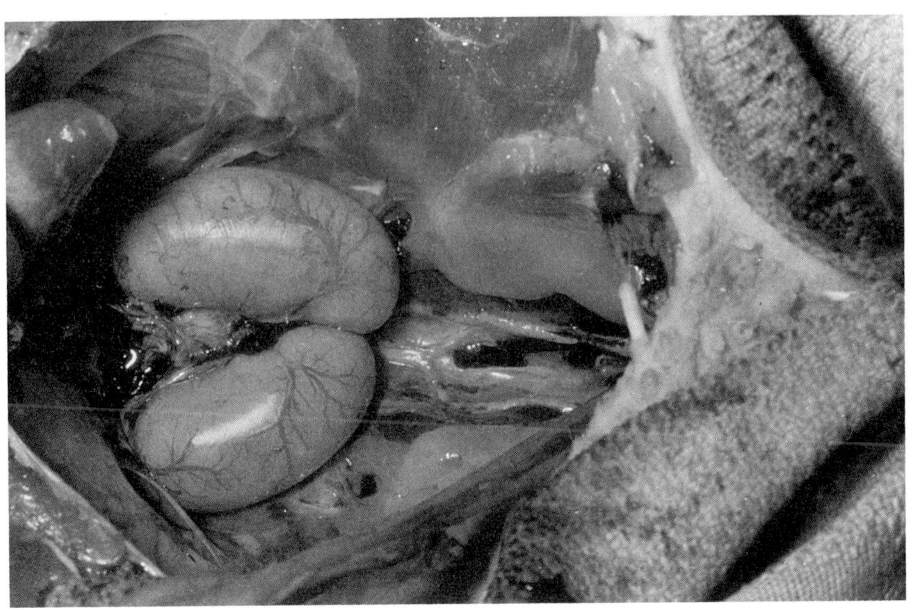

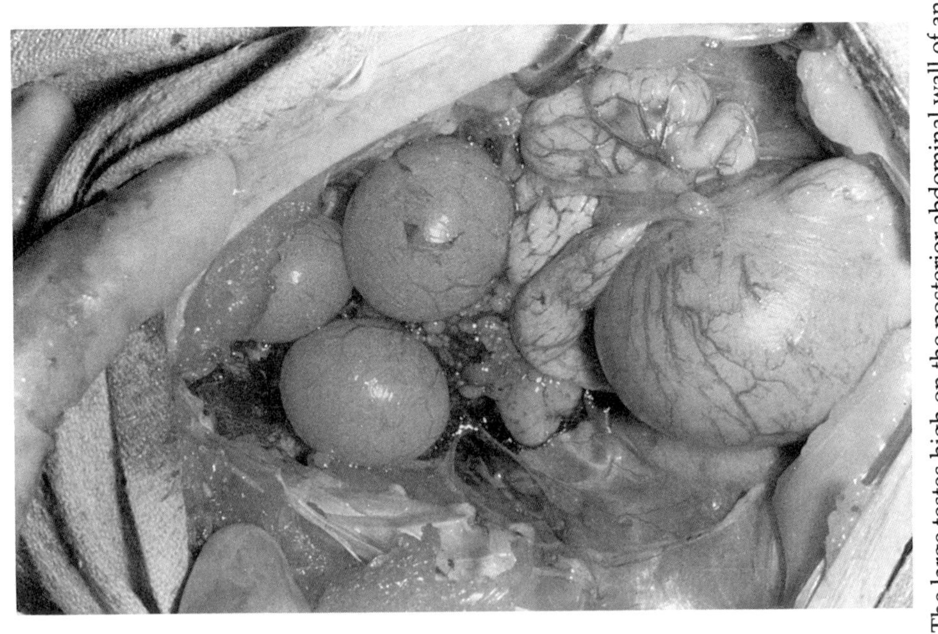

Figure 1.1 the intra-abdominal gonads of the domestic fowl. (a) The large testes high on the posterior abdominal wall of an adult rooster. Note that the testes are larger than the heart, shown at the top of the picture. (b) The single (left) ovary of the hen, showing eggs at various stages of development. The single (left) oviduct contains several eggs in transit.

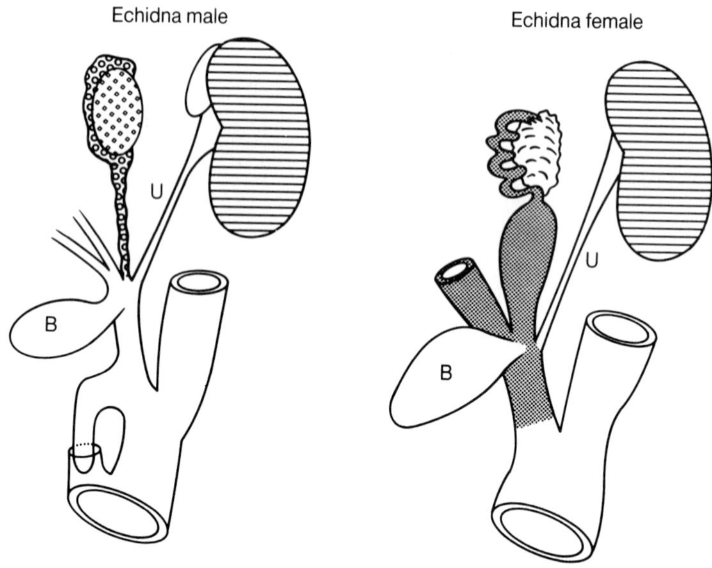

Figure 1.2 Gonadal position in the monotreme echidna. The testes and ovaries are in a similar position near the kidneys. (Redrawn from Reference 41.)

spring the enlarged testes protrude temporarily into sacs near the base of the tail[10] (Figure 1.8). Sloths and armadillos have testes between the bladder and rectum.[11]

The testes of the chinchilla are just inside the inguinal aperture but the caudal epididymis protrudes into a thin-walled scrotal diverticulum[12] (Figure 1.9). Some animals have testes in a subcutaneous pouch which communicates freely with the peritoneum. The southern elephant seal (*Mirounga Leoninia* Linnaeus) has two separate inguinal pouches rather than a single scrotum.[13]

Even where a formed scrotum is present its exact site and degree of development varies widely between species. The hyaena, for instance, has two posterior shallow scrotal pouches,[14] while the kangaroo has a large prepenile scrotum.

In some mammals, the testicular position relative to the scrotum varies with sexual maturity and season. In the bear, for instance, the testes are scrotal from infancy but are held close to the body, except in the adult during the breeding season, when they are pendulous because of scrotal relaxation. The testes of the rhesus macaque descend prenatally into the scrotum, but then re-ascend to the inguinal canal after birth, only to re-enter the scrotum finally at puberty (Figure 1.10).[15]

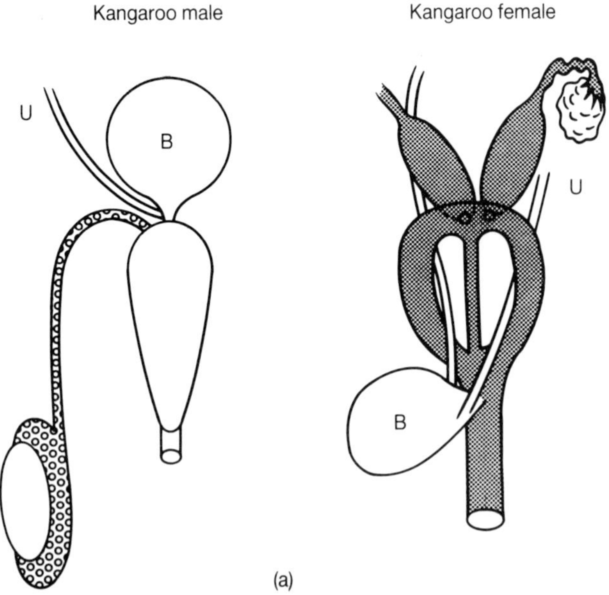

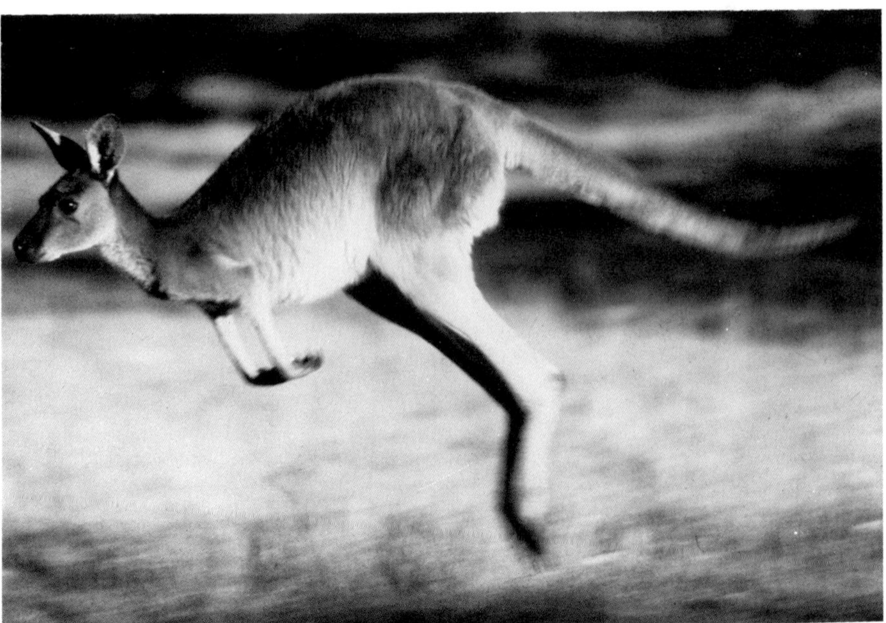

Figure 1.3 Gonadal position in the marsupial (kangaroo). (a) The testis is fully descended into a prepenile scrotum while the ovary remains near the kidney. (Redrawn from Reference 41.) (b) A red kangaroo in full flight. (Kindly provided by Professor MB Renfree.)

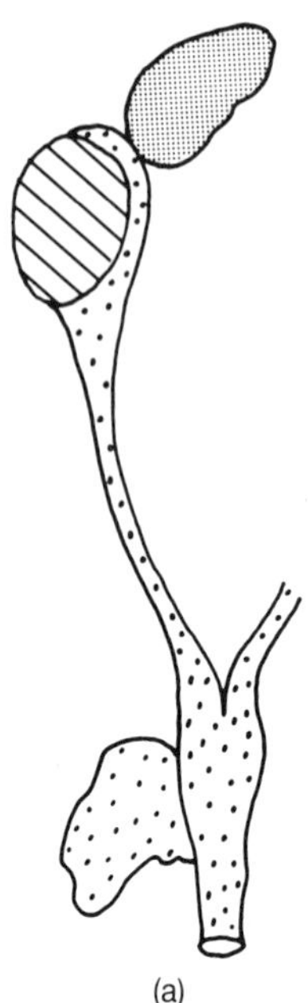

(a)

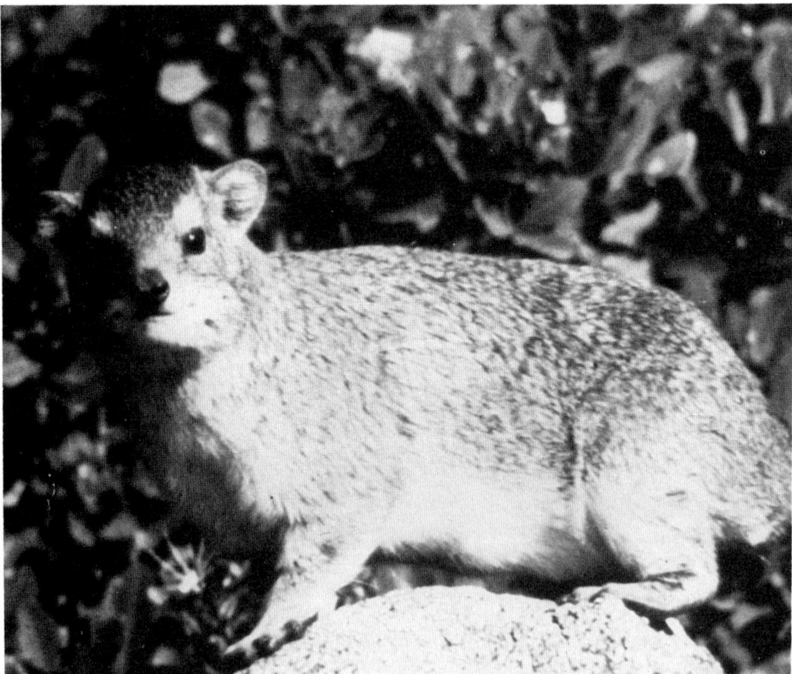

Figure 1.4 (a) The testicular position in the rock hyrax (Reproduced with permission from Reference 4.) (b) The rock hyrax, a small herbivore living in rocky outcrops in parts of Africa.

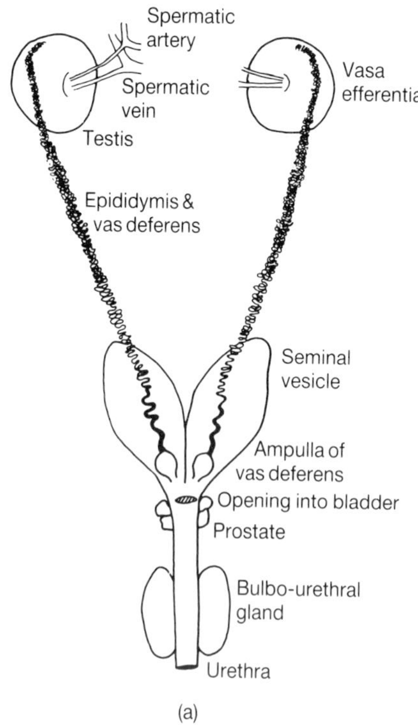

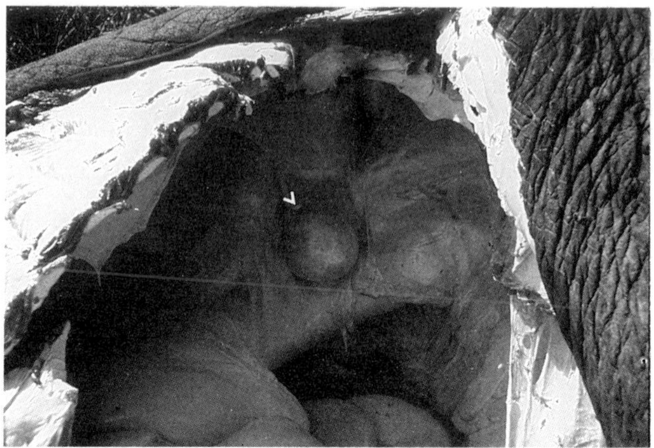

Figure 1.5 (a) The intra-abdominal testes of the African elephant. (Reproduced with permission from Reference 42.) (b) A photograph of a dissection of an African bull elephant showing the large intra-abdominal testis. (Kindly provided by Professor RV Short.)

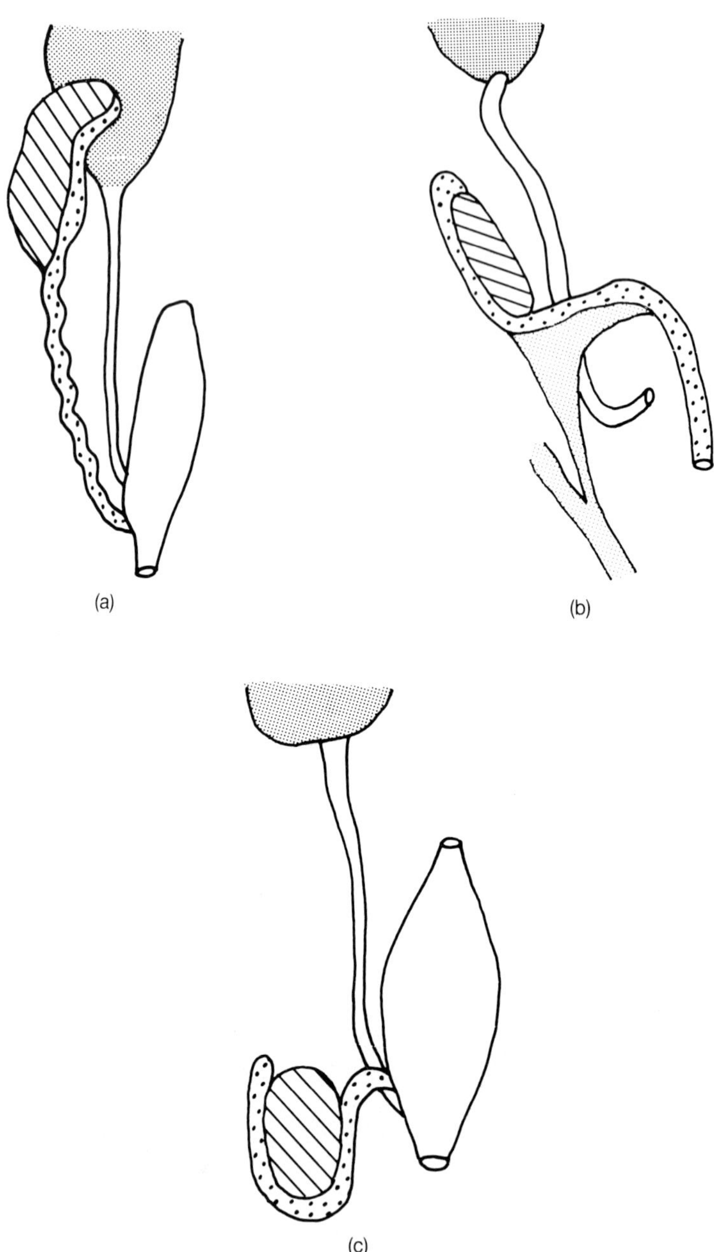

Figure 1.6 Aquatic mammals (Cetaceae), such as (a) the porpoise, (b) the finwhale, or (c) the narwhale, have intra-abdominal testes that have descended to a variable extent. (Reproduced with permission from Reference 4.)

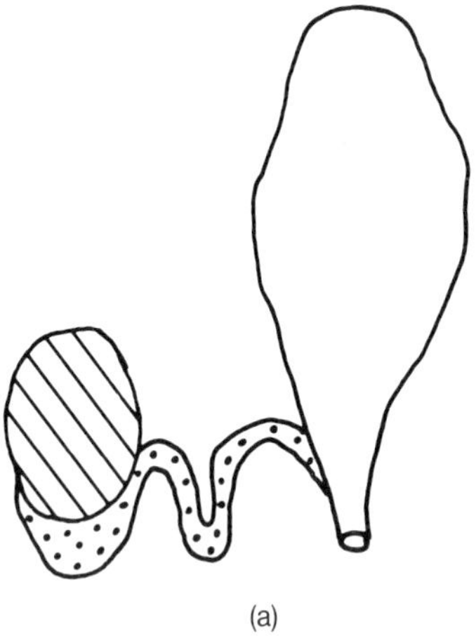

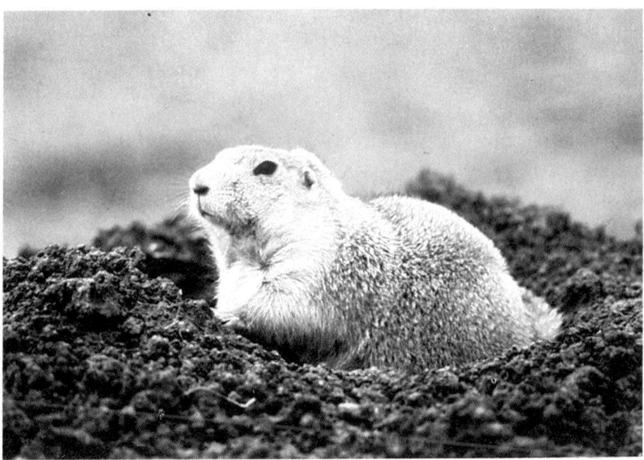

Figure 1.7 (a) The prairie dog has testes that have descended to beside the bladder neck. (b) The prairie dog emerging from its burrow. (Kindly provided by Professor MB Renfree.)

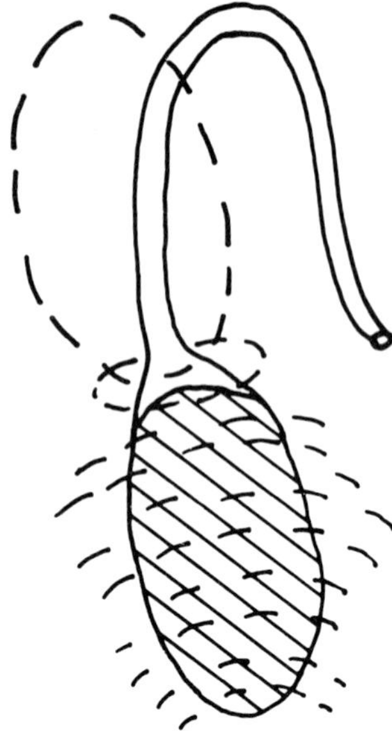

Figure 1.8 The testis of the tree shrew sits inside the inguinal canal, but can descend into a subcutaneous pouch. (Reproduced with permission from Reference 4.)

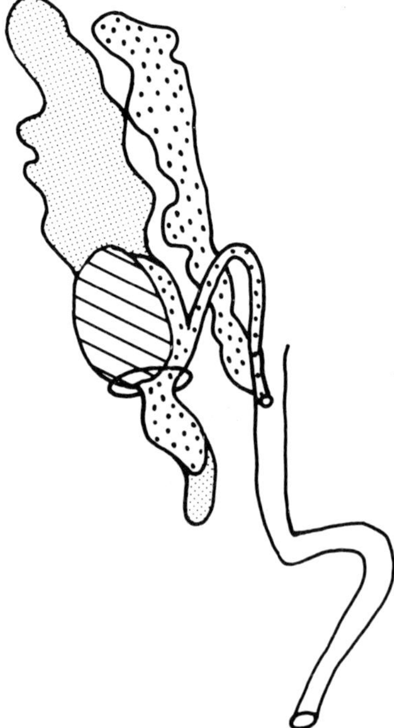

Figure 1.9 The chinchilla's testis is just inside the inguinal ring, but the caudal epididymis protrudes through. (Reproduced with permission from Reference 4.)

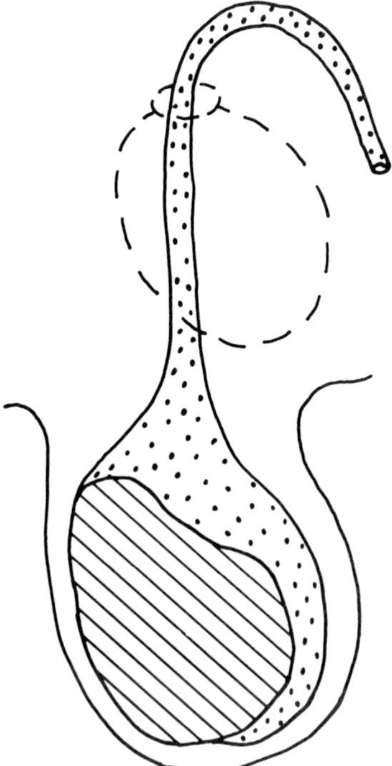

Figure 1.10 The macaque testis descends into a scrotum at birth but then ascends to the groin until puberty, when permanent descent occurs. (Reproduced with permission from Reference 4.)

As can be seen from this brief summary, only a small number of highly specialized mammals have no testicular descent, e.g. monotremes, hyrax, elephant, and possibly some insectivores. Partial intra-abdominal descent occurs in the cetacea (porpoises, dolphins and whales). The testis is inguinal in position in edentates, some insectivores and some ungulates; these animals probably have ancient origins, despite their highly specialized characteristics. Other animals have a subcutaneous pouch rather than a true scrotum, and exhibit periodic or seasonal descent of the testes.

In the large number of modern mammals, e.g. marsupials, ungulates, carnivores and primates, the testes have descended permanently into a definite scrotum (Figure 1.11). While retraction of the testes back into the abdomen is normal in rodents, the processus vaginalis of apes and humans has become obliterated.

During evolution, the testes have migrated from their initial position in the embryonic urogenital ridge, which in most species is revealed in the adult by the position of the ovary. As there are a small number of mammalian species with testes in the same position as the ovary and a large

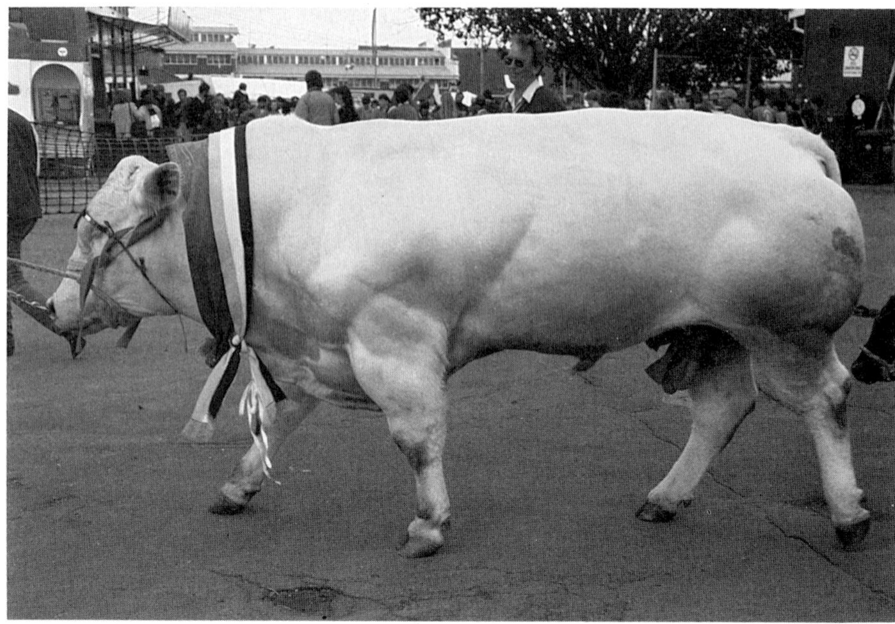

Figure 1.11 The testis in ungulates descends into a pendulous scrotum before birth. In this prize bull the hairless scrotum is quite conspicuous. The studmaster has demonstrated the importance of the scrotum by a prize ribbon.

number with testes in the inguinal region, it would appear that descent to the inguinal region is the first evolutionary phase of descent. These animals probably evolved a mechanism for testicular descent to this point by growth of the gubernaculum.[16] Because the more recently evolved mammals have testes outside the inguinal abdominal wall in a specialized scrotum, we can assume that further descent from the inguinal region offered further evolutionary advantage. In addition, migration of the testis beyond the inguinal region is related to migration of the gubernaculum, which is a process different from the gubernacular enlargement seen in intra-abdominal migration.

1.1.3 Stepwise descent of the testis

The stepwise descent of the testis during mammalian evolution parallels the stepwise descent seen in the modern mammalian fetus, such as the mouse and the human. Between about weeks 10 and 15 of gestation in the human, the testis remains close to the inguinal region because the enlarging gubernaculum in the male acts as an anchor. On the other hand, the gubernaculum in the female fetus remains thin and tenuous, and the ovary shifts away from the inguinal region as the fetus enlarges.[17]

The elongation of the thin gubernaculum in the female is the reverse of the broad, short gubernaculum in the male that remains at a fixed length. After 25–28 weeks, the testis descends rapidly through the inguinal canal, and then migrates more slowly from the external inguinal ring to the scrotum, arriving there at 35–40 weeks. This phase of descent is preceded by migration of the gubernaculum from the inguinal canal to the scrotum.

The stepwise descent of the testis observed in human embryos and laboratory animals led to the concept that testicular descent may occur in two or more phases. This concept was proposed initially by Wensing[18] and more recently by Habenicht and Neumann[19] and ourselves.[20,21] Wensing's observations of the enlargement (or 'swelling reaction') of the male gubernaculum in the pig fetus and other species, coupled with observations of rodents by Habenicht and Neumann,[19] suggested that testicular descent was not only stepwise morphologically, but also stepwise in its apparent control by hormones. The testicular feminizing (TFM) mouse, in which there is a genetic defect in the androgen receptor, provides crucial evidence for stepwise testicular descent because it is unable to respond to circulating androgens.[20] In this animal the swelling reaction of the gubernaculum occurs relatively normally and the testis resides near the inguinal region beside the bladder neck, but no migration outside the abdomen occurs. Our explanation has been that androgens are required for migration from the groin to the scrotum, but that other hormonal factors control intra-abdominal migration and enlargement of the gubernaculum[20] (Figure 1.12).

The detailed modern evidence for multiphasic testicular descent, both morphological and hormonal, is discussed in Chapters 2 and 3: here we summarize some of the historical evidence which has been accumulated over the last two centuries.[3,4]

1.2 Early work on testicular descent

1.2.1 The role of the gubernaculum

The study of testicular descent began in earnest with the observations of John Hunter.[22] In 1762 and 1786 he described the fetal testis and epididymis in the abdomen, and provided the first accurate description of the gubernaculum. He found that the fetal testis was connected to the abdominal wall by a ligament, or 'gubernaculum testis', so-called because it appeared to direct the course of the testis during descent. Hunter thought that the gubernaculum was vascular and fibrous, and covered by fibres of the cremaster muscle.

The relationship between the gubernaculum and the developing cremaster muscle within it was the subject of much controversy, in part related to anatomical differences between species. Seiler[23] described

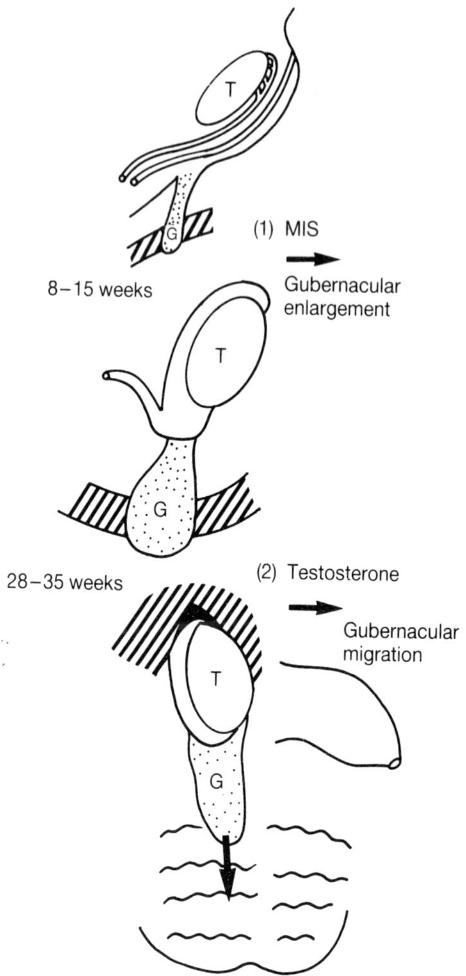

Figure 1.12 Schema showing the two main steps in descent of the human testis (T). Between 8 and 15 weeks, the gubernaculum (G) enlarges in the male. The hormonal regulation of this process remains controversial, although our own proposal is that the regulating hormone is müllerian inhibiting substance (MIS). At 28–35 weeks, the gubernaculum migrates into the scrotum under the control of testosterone.

ascending muscular fibres in the gubernaculum by extrapolation from dissections of adult non-human mammals. Curling[24] described the gubernaculum as a soft, solid cone which varies in shape and size at different stages of descent. He found a bulky central part composed of primitive cellular tissue (i.e. embryonic mesenchyme) surrounded by a layer of muscular fibres and another layer of 'mesenchyme', the whole being invested by peritoneum except posteriorly. Cloquet[25] and Carus[26] believed that the cremaster was formed mechanically from the passage of the testis through the abdominal wall, which pulled loops of muscle fibres off the conjoint tendon made up of the internal oblique and transversus abdominus muscles.

Migration of the gubernaculum from the inguinal region to the scrotum was well recognized in the nineteenth century. Cleland[27] dissected human fetuses of 5 and 6 months' gestation and found that the fetal gubernaculum ended in the inguinal abdominal wall, and did not extend directly from the testis to the scrotum. Hence the alternative name for the gubernaculum became the genito-inguinal ligament. Cleland believed that the gubernaculum migrated ahead of the testis into the scrotum, creating a space lined by peritoneum. He did not think that the cremaster muscle pulled the testis into the scrotum.

One theory which was popularized by Lockwood[28] was that differential growth of the posterior abdominal wall relative to the pelvis meant that the testis remained stationary while its surroundings grew further apart. Lockwood did not believe that the gubernaculum contracted, but imagined that the gubernaculum passively held the testis near the inguinal region. In recent years, this passive effect of relative growth has been interpreted to mean that this phase of descent is unimportant. However, anchoring of the gonad by the gubernaculum fails to occur in the female fetus, indicating that this effect in the male is likely to be hormonally mediated. In fact, in the female fetus the ovary actually ascends relative to the position it occupied initially in relation to the inguinal region.

Lockwood also believed that the gubernacular muscle must serve some purpose, leading to the idea that the different final location to the testis may be caused by a fan-shaped gubernaculum. Although he was unable to demonstrate these so-called 'tails of Lockwood' on dissection, he postulated their existence as an explanation for the observation that the gubernaculum migrates into a range of different positions (Figure 1.13).[29] On the other hand, Coley[30] and Sebileau[31] did not believe that an ectopic position of the testis was caused by an aberrant gubernaculum. Many surgeons and authors believe that an undescended testis or ectopic testis is caused by mechanical obstruction.[32–34]

1.2.2 The role of hormones

In the early twentieth century the advent of hormonal studies of sexual development undermined the credibility of previously held mechanical and anatomical concepts.[35,36] In an effort to 'explain' testicular descent in endocrinological terms, these earlier mechanical hypotheses were discarded. Initially, the simplest hormonal concept was that male androgens under pituitary control caused testicular descent.[37] This led to attempts to treat boys with undescended testis with crude preparations of human chorionic gonadotrophin and, once these steroids had been

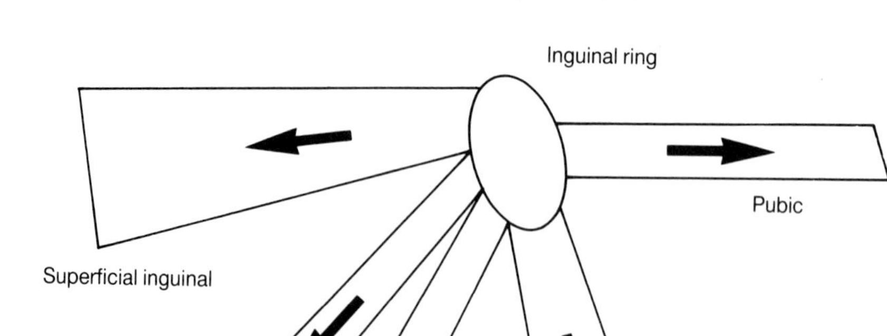

Figure 1.13 Schema showing the gubernacular 'tails of Lockwood'. (Reproduced with permission from Reference 3.)

synthesized, with androgens. Early optimistic reports of success of these treatments were eventually replaced with more realistic and consistently disappointing reports.

1.2.3 Phasic control

Experimental evidence from the fetus has failed to support the idea that testicular descent is controlled by testicular androgens alone.[18,19] Such discrepancies have eventually led to the proposal of multihormonal control.[16]

Recent evidence from our own laboratory suggests that testicular descent occurs in two separate phases, each of which is controlled by different hormones (see Figure 1.12).[39] Current debate focuses on which hormones are involved and how they mediate their action.[39,40] The evidence for and against these various hypotheses is discussed in Chapters 2 and 3.

References

1. Bedford JM. Anatomical evidence for the epididymis as the prime mover in the evolution of the scrotum. *Am J Anat* 1978; **152:** 483–508.
2. Grant T. *The Platypus*, Sydney: NSW University Press, 1984: pp 40–1.

3. Williams MPL, Hutson JM. The history of ideas about testicular descent. *Pediatr Surg Int* 1991a; **6:** 180–4.
4. Williams MPL, Hutson JM. The phylogeny of testicular descent. *Pediatr Surg Int* 1991b; **6:** 162–6.
5. Short RV. Reproductive Patterns. In: Austin CR, Short RV, eds. *Reproduction in Mammals* (Book 4) Cambridge: Cambridge University Press, pp.1–33, 1972.
6. Glover TD, Sale JB. The reproductive system of male rock hyrax (*Procavia* and *Heterohyrax*) *J Zool Lond* 1968; **156:** 351–62.
7. Chi Ping. On the testis and its accessory structures in the porpoise. *Anat Rec* 1926; **32:** 113–7.
8. Meek A. The reproductive organs of cetacea. *J Anat* 1918; **52:** 186–210.
9. Anthony A. Seasonal reproductive cycle in the normal and experimentally treated male prairie dog, *cynomus ludovicianus*. *J Morphol* 1953; **93:** 331–69.
10. Marshall FHA. The male generative cycle in the hedgehog; with experiments on the functional correlation between the essential and accessory sexual organs. *J Physiol* 1911; **43:** 247–60.
11. Wislocki GB. Observations on the gross and microscopic anatomy of the sloths (*Bradpus griseus grisues* Gray and *choloepus hoffmanni* Peters). *J Morph* 1928; **46:** 317.
12. Roos TB, Schackelford RM. Some observations on the gross anatomy of the genital system and two endocrine organs and body weights in the chinchilla. *Anat Rec* 1965; **123:** 301–11.
13. Bryden MM. Testicular temperature in the southern elephant seal, *Mirounga Leonina* (Linn). *J Reprod Fertil* 1967; **13:** 583–4.
14. Matthews LH. Reproduction in the spotted hyaena, *Crocuta crocuta* (Ernleben). *Phil Trans B Roy Soc*, 1941; 230.
15. Miller RA. The inguinal canal of primates. *Am J Anat* 1947; **80:** 117–42.
16. Wensing CJG, Colenbrander B. Normal and abnormal testicular descent. *Oxf Rev Reprod Biol* 1986; **8:** 131–64.
17. Jirasek JE. Genital ducts and external genitalia: development and anomalies. *Birth Defects* 1971; **7:** 131–9.
18. Wensing CJG. Testicular descent in some domestic mammals III Search for the factors that regulate the gubernacular reaction. *Proc Kon Ned Akad Wetensch C* 1973; **76:** 196–202.
19. Habenicht UF, Neumann F. 1983 Hormonal regulation of testicular descent. *Adv Anat Embryol Cell Biol* 1983; **81:** 1–54.
20. Hutson JM. A biphasic model for the hormonal control of testicular descent. *Lancet* 1985; **i:** 419–21.
21. Hutson JM. Testicular feminization: a model for testicular descent in mice and men. *J Ped Surg* 1986; **21:** 195–8.
22. Hunter J. A description of the situation of the testis in the foetus, with its descent into the scrotum. In: *Observations on certain parts of the animal oeconomy*. London, 1786, pp. 1–26.
23. Seiler BW. *Observations nonnules de testiculorum ex abdomine in scrotum descensus et partium genitalium anomalis*. Leipzig, 1817.
24. Curling JB. Observations on the structure of the gubernaculum and on the descent of the testis in the foetus. *Lancet* 1841; **ii:** 70–4.
25. Cloquet J. *Recherches Anatomique sur les Hernies de l'Abdomen*, Paris, 1817.
26. Carus CG. *An Introduction to the Comparative Anatomy of Animals*. London. 1827: Vol. 2, p. 346.
27. Cleland J. *The Mechanism of the Gubernaculum Testis*, Prize Thesis. Edinburgh: MacLachlan & Stewart, 1856.
28. Lockwood CB. Development and transition of the testis, normal and abnormal. *J Anat Physiol* 1888; **22:** 505–41.

29. McGregor AL. The third inguinal ring. *Surg Gynecol Obstet* 1929; **49:** 273–307.
30. Coley WB. The treatment of the undescended or maldescended testis associated with inguinal hernia. *Ann Surg* 1908; **48:** 321–50.
31. Sebileau. *Les Envelopes du Testicule.* Paris, 1897.
32. Bertelsen A, Thorup J, Pedersen PV, Mauritzen, Skakkebaek N. Intravenous LH-RH treatment of cryptorchidism. *Eur J Pediatr* 1987; **146 [Suppl 2]:** 540–1.
33. De Muinck Kiezer-Schrama SMPF, Hazebroek FWJ, Matroos AW *et al.* Double blind, placebo-controlled study of luteinising-hormone-releasing-hormone nasal spray in treatment of undescended testes. *Lancet* 1986; **i:** 876–80.
34. Scorer CG. The anatomy of testicular descent – normal and incomplete. *Br J Surg* 1972; **49:** 357–67.
35. Engle ET. Experimentally induced descent of the testis in the Macacus Monkey by hormones from the anterior pituitary and pregnancy urine. *Endocrinology* 1932; **16:** 513–20.
36. Lillie FR. The theory of the freemartin. *Science* 1916; **43:** 611–3.
37. Hamilton JB. The effect of male hormone on descent of the testis. *Anat Rec* 1938; **70:** 533–41.
38. Hutson JM, Donahoe PK. The hormonal control of testicular descent. *Endocrin Rev.* 1986; **7:** 270–83.
39. Hadziselimovic F. Histology and ultrastructure of normal and cryptorchid testes. In: Hadziselimovic F. ed. *Cryptorchidism, Management and Implications.* Berlin: Springer-Verlag, 1983, pp. 35–58.
40. Hutson JM, Williams MPL, Fallat ME, Attah A. Testicular descent: new insights into its hormonal control. *Oxford Rev Reprod Biol* 1990; **12:** 1–56.
41. Renfree MB. Ontogeny, genetic control and phylogeny of female reproduction in monotreme and therian mammals. In: Szalay FS, Novacek MJ, McKenna MC, eds. *Mammalian Phylogeny,* New York: Springer-Verlag, 1992.
42. Short RV, Mann T, Hay MF. Male reproductive organs of the African elephant, *Loxodonta africana. J Reprod Fertil* 1967; **13:** 517–36.

2

Transabdominal migration of the testis

2.1 The first phase of descent

Since the 1930s testicular descent has been thought to be controlled by androgens (Figure 2.1a). In the last 20 years, however, opinions have begun to diverge about the role of androgens and recent evidence suggests that androgens may have little or no role to play in the initial transabdominal migration of the testes.[1,2]

Early studies produced apparently contradictory observations because it was assumed that testicular descent occurred in one step. Wensing and colleagues [3] studied early events in the fetal pig and dog, and were unable to find a convincing role for androgens in testicular descent, whereas those looking at later events with postnatal rats found androgens had a significant effect.[4,5] Another animal model which was used extensively was the male fetal mouse exposed to oestrogen.[6–10] The fetal mouse studies showed that oestrogen inhibited not only androgen production by the testis, but also testicular descent and regression of the Müllerian ducts. The results were interpreted as supporting a role for androgens in testicular descent, although other conclusions are feasible, as are discussed later in this chapter.

The contradictory conclusions arising from these different model systems led to the proposal that testicular descent may in fact occur in two phases rather than one, each phase being under separate hormonal control (Figure 2.1b).[1,11,12]

The first phase involves transabdominal descent of the testis; a common feature of which is enlargement of the gubernaculum, now known as the 'swelling reaction'. Gubernacular enlargement has been linked closely to transabdominal migration of the testis.[13]

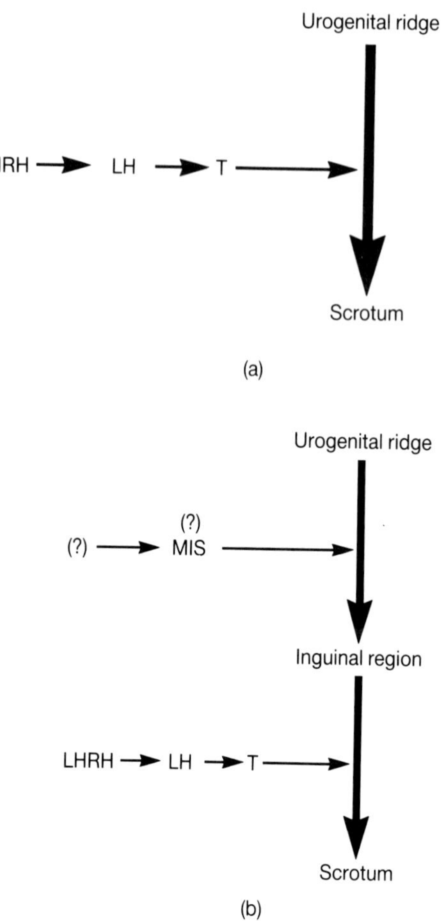

Figure 2.1 (a) The first endocrinological hypothesis to account for testicular descent. Testicular testosterone (T) was stimulated via the hypothalamus (LHRH) and pituitary (LH) to induce complete descent. (b) The two-step endocrinological hypothesis which proposes that testicular descent occurs in two morphologically distinct phases. Control of the first step is unknown, with our own hypothesis being that müllerian inhibiting substance (MIS) is the active agent. The second step is controlled by androgens analagously to the original hypothesis.

2.2 The gubernacular 'swelling reaction'

In the late 1960s Wensing began a detailed study of the gubernaculum using the pig fetus as a model. He found that enlargement and outgrowth of the caudal end of the gubernaculum was associated with early transabdominal migration of the testis.[14] Similarly in the mouse, the testis has been observed to move relatively closer to the groin between 15 and

17 days of gestation.[8] This relative movement of the gonad does not occur in the female fetus, where the ovary maintains a constant relationship to the lumbar region (Figure 2.2) and may even appear to ascend in the abdominal cavity relative to the inguinal region. The gubernaculum of the female has no swelling reaction, but rather remains thin and cord-like, with elongation of this cord in proportion to fetal enlargement (Figure 2.2)

In the male, the enlarged gubernaculum anchors the testis close to the inguinal region as the embryo enlarges. The distance between the testis and the inguinal region remains fairly constant when measured in millimetres, but appears to shorten when compared with the distance between the ovary and the inguinal region. Previously, the change in testicular position had been interpreted as indicating a merely passive role for the gubernaculum,[15,16] when this may be the opposite to the actual situation.

The gubernacular swelling reaction is caused by cell division within the fetal gubernaculum, as well as deposition of a significant amount of extra-cellular matrix.[17,18] This extra-cellular matrix is primarily hyaluronic acid and chondroitin sulphate.[19] These matrix molecules are particularly hydrophilic and lead to significant absorption of water into the

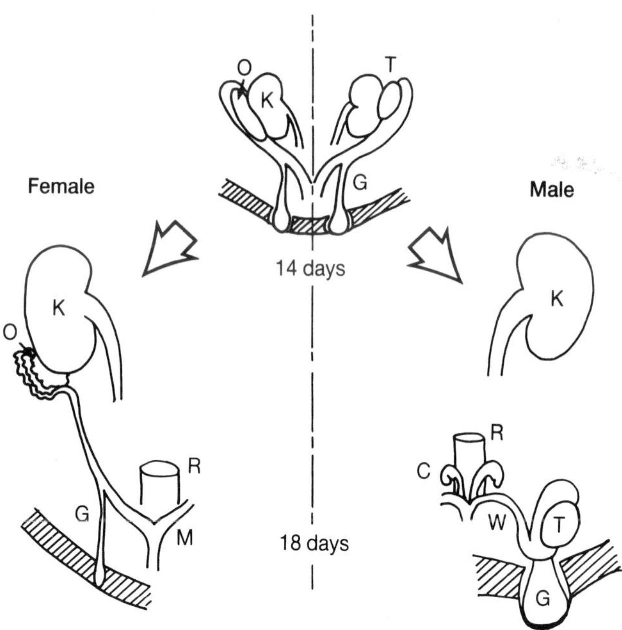

Figure 2.2 Schema showing the relative movements of the ovary (O) and testis (T) in the fetal mouse between 14 and 18 days of gestation (K, kidney; G, gubernaculum; C, coagulating glands; M, müllerian ducts; W, wolffian ducts; R, rectum). (Reproduced with permission from Reference 32.)

gubernaculum, giving it an appearance similar to the Wharton's jelly found in the umbilical cord. This swelling reaction is unaffected by experimental manipulation of fetal androgen levels. Injection of androgens into the rat or pig fails to stimulate the gubernacular reaction in fetal females,[13] while androgen replacement after orchidectomy does not prevent gubernacular atrophy in the fetal dog.[20,21] Perhaps the most telling evidence against a role for androgens comes from animals with complete androgen resistance (testicular feminization syndrome). In the fetal pig, raccoon dog, mouse and human with complete androgen resistance, the gubernacular swelling reaction and transabdominal testicular descent remains essentially normal (Figure 2.3).[22–24] In these animals with a mutation in the androgen receptor which prevents androgen action, the swelling reaction and the gonadal position are initially normal for the male (Figure 2.4). Further evidence that androgens are not involved in the swelling reaction comes from experiments using the synthetic

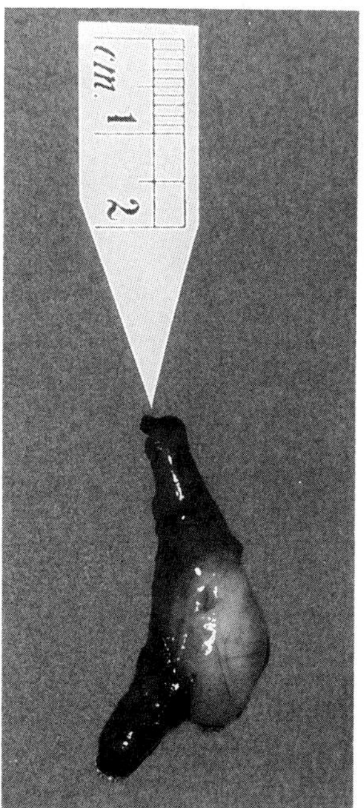

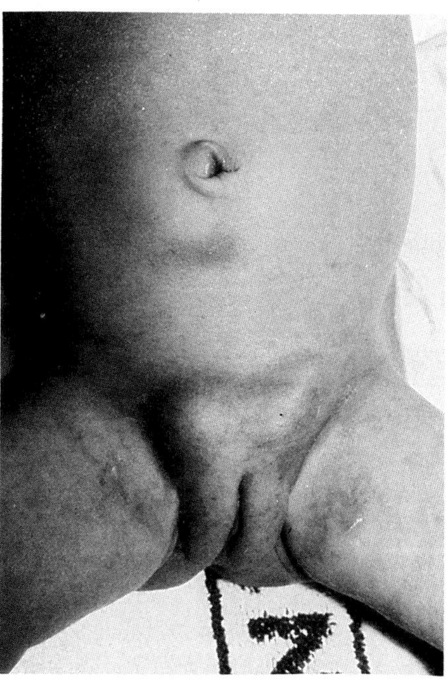

Figure 2.3 (a) A testis and gubernaculum excised from a human with complete androgen resistance. Despite absence of androgen receptors (and hence no epididymal development), the gubernaculum has undergone a normal 'swelling reaction'.
(b) One-week-old genetic male with complete androgen resistance and normal female phenotype. The transabdominal migration of the testes is normal, but inguino-scrotal migration is absent, leaving the testes in the groin. (Reproduced with permission from Reference 32.)

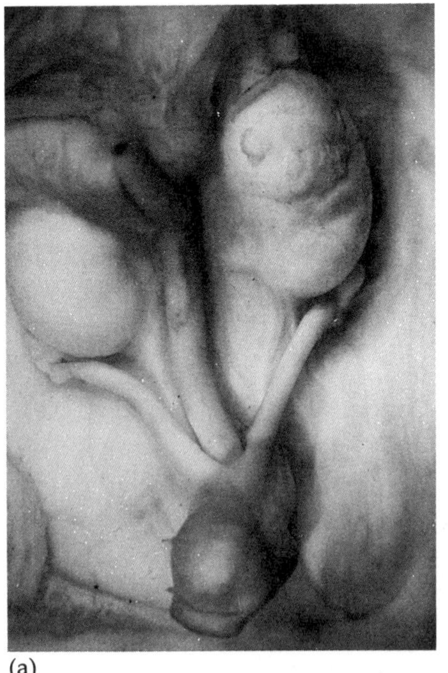
(a)

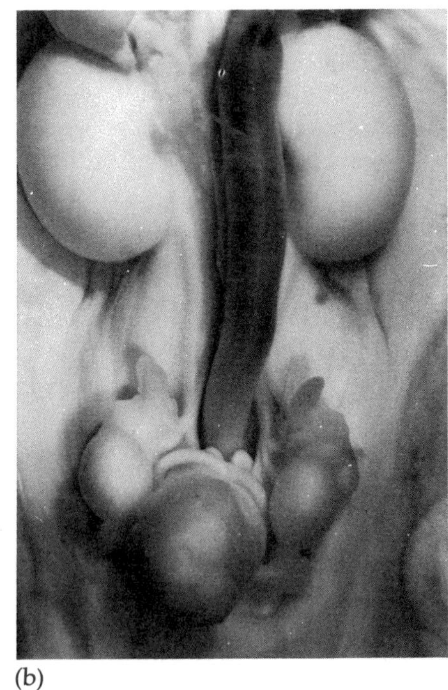
(b)

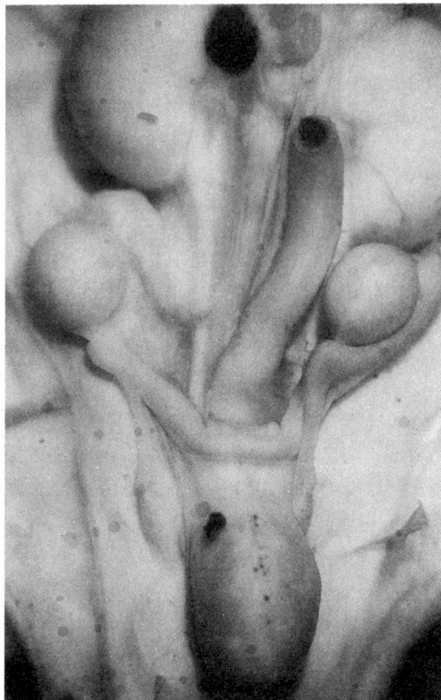
(c)

Figure 2.4 (a) Normal anatomy of a female mouse at birth. The ovaries are located just behind the lower poles of the kidneys. (Reproduced with permission from Reference 35.) (b) Normal male mouse at birth, after completion of transabdominal descent but before inguinoscrotal migration occurs. The testes are located beside the bladder neck. (c) Oestrogen-treated male mouse at birth. The testes remain high in the abdomen and the müllerian ducts are preserved. (Reproduced from Reference 31.)

anti-androgen, cyproterone acetate: when it is injected into fetal rats the transabdominal phase of descent is not affected.[11,25]

Some recent authors have proposed that androgens may still have a role in gubernacular swelling, despite the contrary evidence cited above. Husmann and McPhaul[26] have identified androgen receptors in the mesenchymal core of the gubernaculum in fetal rats, but their maximum expression is between days 18 and 21, which is after the swelling reaction is almost complete in this animal. Androgen receptors have been found also in the gubernaculum of the fetal pig,[27] but both the receptor binding affinity and its capacity were significantly lower than in known androgen-sensitive target tissues (e.g. prostate). Spencer *et al.*[28] have shown that the anti-androgen, flutamide, given between days 15 and 17 of gestation of a rat, can prevent testicular descent at 28 days after birth. There was some hypoplasia of the gubernacular swelling reaction (about 20%) but the testes were nearly all descended through the inguinal canal, confirming that transabdominal descent was not interrupted significantly. These studies were interpreted as supporting a role for androgens in transabdominal descent although, in our view, they merely confirm that transabdominal descent does not need androgen stimulation.

2.3 Oestrogen-treated mouse

As experimental studies using fetal models and animals with complete androgen resistance showed, transabdominal migration of the testis did not require androgens. However, the oestrogen-treated mouse remained a major stumbling block because this experimental model had been used to support a role for androgens in descent.[8] Fetal male mice exposed to exogenous oestrogen were observed to have undescended testes, the degree of which was directly related to the degree of atrophy of the Wolffian duct and the mesonephros, which suggested suppression of androgen-dependent development.[29] Hadziselimovic[30] found low levels of serum androgens at birth after fetal male mice were exposed to oestrogens. He postulated that this suppression by oestrogen was caused by negative feedback on the hypothalamic–pituitary axis, and that this suppression led to depressed androgen production by the testis and subsequent inhibition of testicular descent. Simultaneous treatment with human chorionic gonadotrophin (hCG) at the time of oestrogen injection caused a rise in serum androgen levels,[30] supporting the contention that oestrogen caused a defect by suppression of androgen secretion.

The oestrogen-treated mouse was a key model for understanding transabdominal descent, since it appeared to give contradictory results from those seen in untreated mice and other models with complete androgen resistance. Because of its central role in understanding this phase, we have studied this model closely. First, we showed that injection of oestrogen into pregnant mice caused complete lack of testicular descent in male offspring, with the testis located at the lower pole of the kidney (Figure 2.4).[31,32] When human chorionic gonadotrophin was injected simultaneously with oestrogen prenatally the circulating androgen levels were not inhibited as much as with oestrogen alone, but the position of the testis remained completely undescended.[31,32] Secondly, when testicular feminizing male mice were exposed to oestrogen *in utero*, they also demonstrated complete lack of descent of the testis, while in normal TFM mice the testis had descended to a position beside the bladder neck by birth (Figure 2.5).[10] Similar results were obtained after oestrogen exposure in the mutant hypogonadal mouse.[33]

A striking feature of the fetal mouse exposed to oestrogen is the abnormal persistence of the müllerian ducts in genetic males.[6] The close association between müllerian duct retention and undescended testes in mice exposed to oestrogen has been explained by Josso as being caused simply by the müllerian duct mechanically preventing

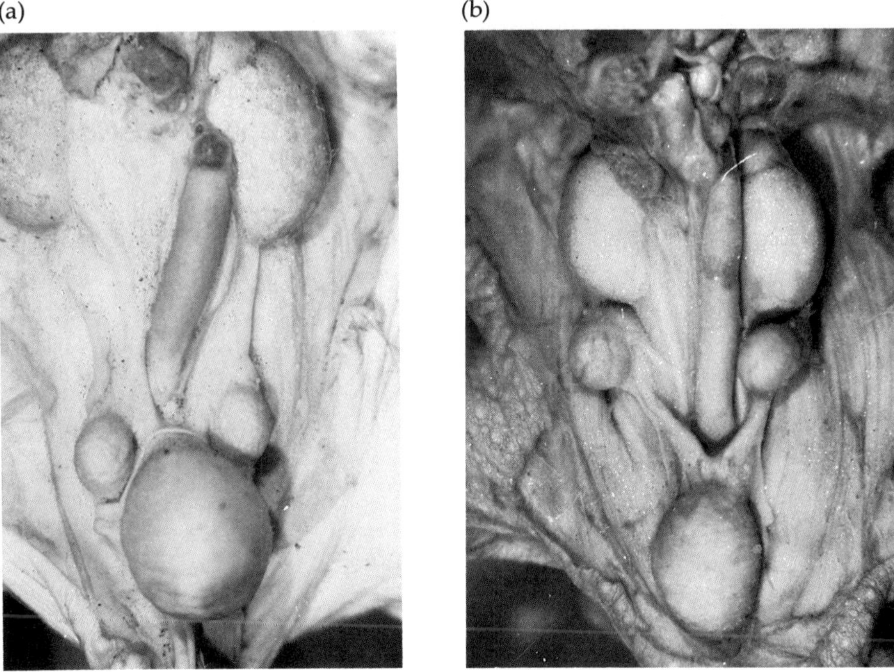

Figure 2.5 (a) Untreated neonatal mouse with complete androgen resistance, showing the testes in the normal position beside the bladder neck. Note the absence of the epididymis, vas and coagulating glands (rodent equivalent of seminal vesicles). (b) Neonatal mouse with complete androgen resistance exposed to oestradiol benzoate *in utero*. The testes are located immediately below the kidneys and the müllerian ducts are retained. (Reproduced with permission from Reference 10.)

testicular descent.[34] To determine whether müllerian duct retention was the cause of undescent, as distinct from an associated effect of oestrogen, we injected pregnant mice with oestrogen on day fifteen of gestation, after regression of the müllerian duct. Oestrogen still caused undescended testis at birth, even though the müllerian duct was represented by only a few vestigial cysts.[35] This experiment suggested that oestrogen blocked testicular descent directly, and since the gubernaculum is atrophic in response to oestrogen[36] it is consistent with the hypothesis that oestrogen prevents the gubernacular swelling reaction.

Our studies of the oestrogen-treated fetal mouse have led us to the hypothesis that oestrogen has a primary effect of inhibiting the swelling reaction of the gubernaculum, as well as a second primary effect of inhibiting müllerian duct regression (Figure 2.6). Since the latter is controlled by müllerian inhibiting substance (MIS),[37] we postulated that oestrogens might suppress the effect of müllerian inhibiting substance not only on the müllerian duct, but also on the gubernaculum. Support for an action of oestrogen in inhibiting this role of MIS has been documented in the chicken embryo and the mouse embryo, where exposure to oestrogen protects the müllerian duct against MIS action.[9,38,39]

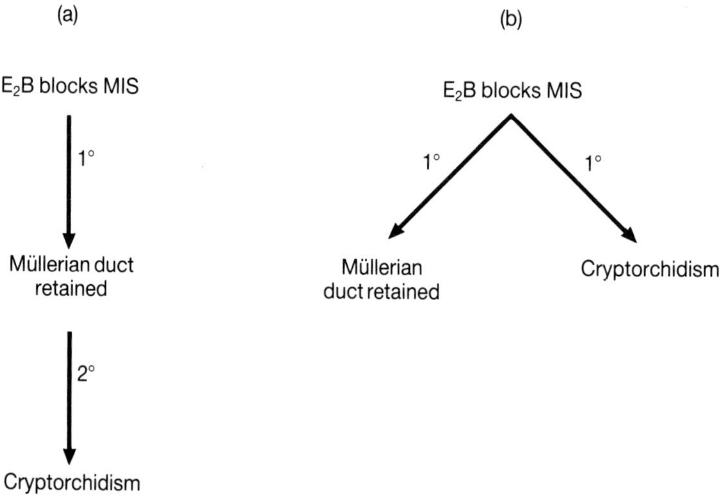

Figure 2.6 The two hypotheses proposed to account for the combination of müllerian duct retention and cryptorchidism in mice treated with oestradiol benzoate. Hypothesis (A) proposes that cryptorchidism is secondary to 'mechanical drag' by the retained ducts, whereas (B) proposes direct inhibition of descent by oestradiol. The latter hypothesis was supported by Luthra and Hutson[35] 1990. (Reproduced with permission from reference 35.)

2.4 Persistent müllerian duct syndrome

Compelling evidence that transabdominal testicular descent is controlled by MIS comes from the rare clinical disorder of persistent müllerian duct syndrome. This is a genetic abnormality of MIS secretion or its putative receptor. Patients have normal male external genitalia, but completely retained müllerian ducts (fallopian tubes, uterus and upper vagina) as well as totally undescended testes.[40–42] Human males with this abnormality have testes in a pseudo-ovarian position (Figure 2.7), as has also been reported in the bull.[43] The status of the gubernaculum in this syndrome is not documented adequately, but detailed case reports of this syndrome have consistently failed to describe any gubernacular structures. In addition, not only is cryptorchidism present in most cases, but an extremely rare abnormality of testicular position, transverse testicular ectopia, is present in 10% of these patients.[44] Both testes are in the same inguinal hernial sac, and neither testis appears to be anchored to

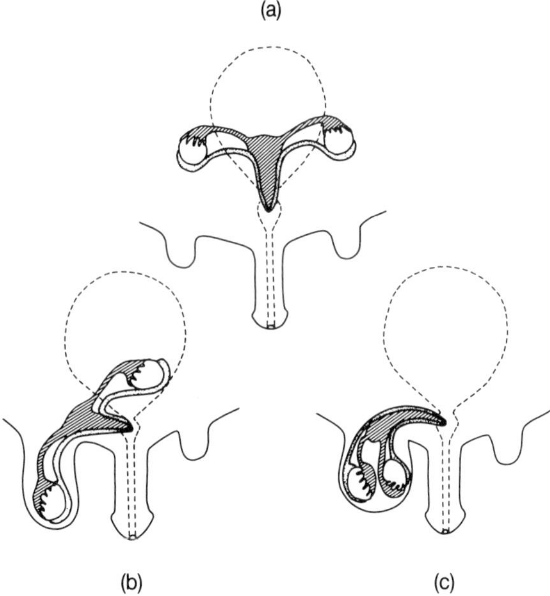

Figure 2.7 The three clinical presentations of persistent müllerian duct syndrome. (a) The majority (60–70%) of patients have testes in the normal position of ovaries, and the inguinal hernial sacs remain empty. (b) A smaller group (20–30%) have one testis in an inguinal hernia or the scrotum along with its attached tube and uterus. This is known as 'hernia uteri inguinalis'. (c) About 10% of patients have both testes herniated into one processus vaginalis (transverse testicular ectopia). (Reproduced with permission from Reference 44.)

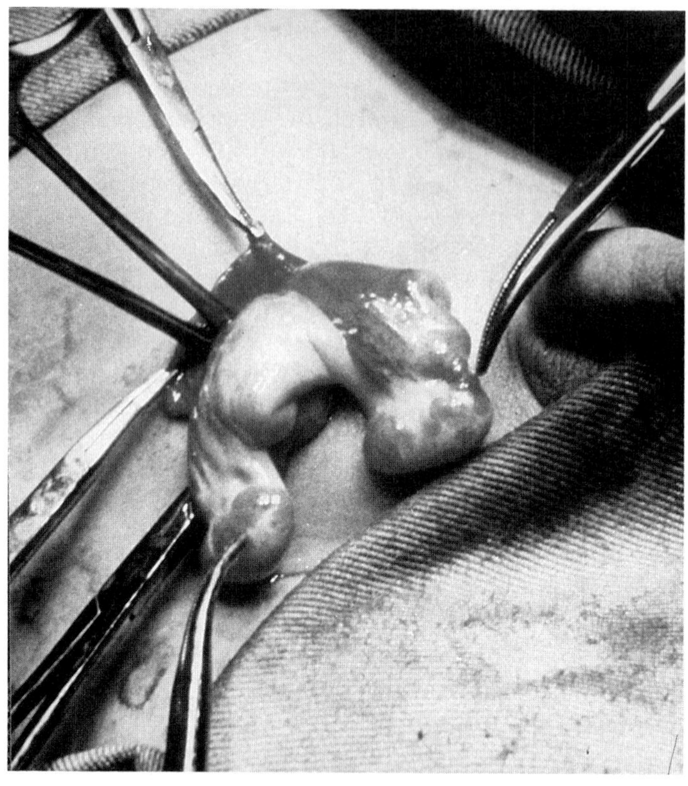

Figure 2.8 A boy with persistent müllerian duct syndrome and transverse testicular ectopia. Operative photograph showing both testes and the uterus and tubes in a right inguinal hernia. Note the lack of gubernacular attachments. (Reproduced with permission from Reference 44.)

the inguinal region by a gubernacular structure (Figure 2.8). In addition, there is no evidence of the round ligaments, ligaments of the ovary, or male gubernacular attachments.

In persistent müllerian duct syndrome there is lack of transabdominal testicular descent, a deficiency of the gubernaculum, and complete retention of the müllerian ducts. These features all point to müllerian inhibiting substance having a major role in stimulating the gubernacular swelling reaction (and, hence transabdominal testicular descent) as well as müllerian duct regression. The strong association in this syndrome between the degree of müllerian duct regression and the degree of gubernacular development and testicular descent is seen also in other types of ambiguous genitalia: in male pseudohermaphrodites from other causes where the testis is dysplastic (Figure 2.9), the degree of müllerian duct retention is directly related to the degree of gonadal descent.[45]

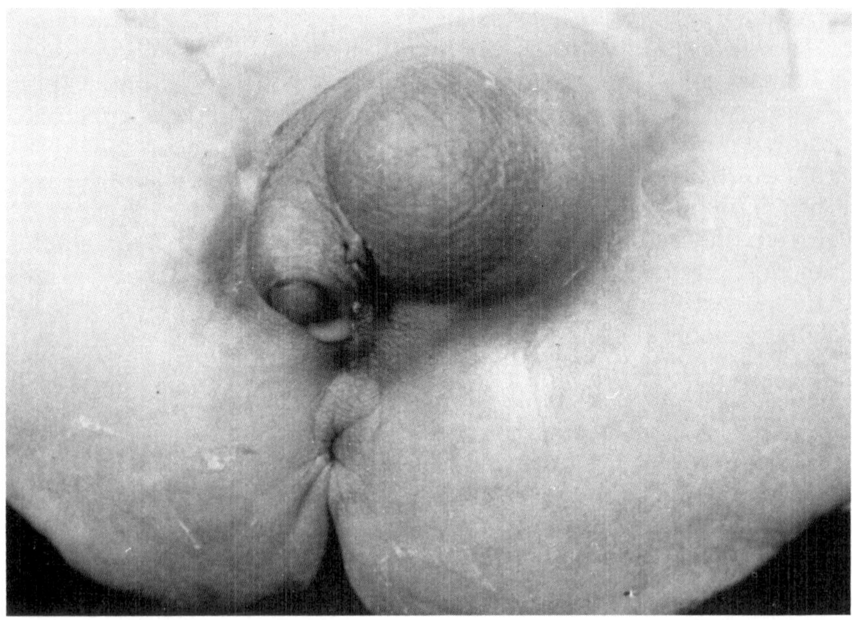

Figure 2.9 The external genitalia of a male pseudohermaphrodite with gonadal dysplasia (mixed gonadal dysgenesis). On the left side the gonadal development is less affected, with some local secretion of testosterone and müllerian inhibiting substance: the testis has descended and the ipsilateral müllerian duct has regressed. The right gonad is completely dysplastic ('streak' gonad) and has failed to descend at all. The adjacent müllerian duct is retained. Note the vaginal mucus (stimulated by maternal hormones) at the opening of the urogenital sinus.

2.5 The role of müllerian inhibiting substance (MIS)

The link between müllerian duct regression and the gubernacular swelling reaction points to a role for MIS, but there are some contradictory results. In pregnant rabbits, immunization against purified bovine MIS (also known as 'anti-müllerian hormone') failed to cause undescended testes in male offspring, despite retention of the müllerian ducts in these males.[46] Another experiment suggesting that MIS is not involved in gubernacular enlargement has been reported by Fentener van Vlissingen *et al.*[23] where purified bovine MIS failed to stimulate cell division in pig gubernacular fibroblasts maintained in tissue culture. By contrast, a low molecular weight dialysate of testicular extract stimulated gubernacular cell division. They have named this low molecular weight substance as 'descendin'.

At present it is difficult to reconcile those studies that fail to demonstrate a role for MIS with the results of the oestrogen-treated mouse and the human mutation of persistent müllerian duct syndrome. To test the role of MIS directly, we have exposed fetal mouse gubernacula to human recombinant MIS (kindly donated by Professor Patricia K Donahoe), that has been highly purified from a Chinese hamster ovary cell line. Gubernacula maintained in organ culture and exposed to MIS enlarge secondary to deposition of extra-cellular matrix and some mitosis (Attah *et al.*, unpublished observations). This preliminary result suggests that human recombinant MIS is capable of inducing the gubernacular swelling reaction in organ culture. The relationship of this experiment to the pig gubernacular fibroblasts in tissue culture maintained by Fentener van Vlissingen[47] remains uncertain, but it may be that the latter work has identified a proteolytic fragment of MIS which stimulates gubernacular cell division. Further studies will be necessary to resolve the role of müllerian inhibiting substance in the gubernacular swelling reaction.

2.6 Conclusion

The evidence that testicular descent occurs in at least two steps is now well established. The gubernaculum appears to be the prime mediator of the first phase of descent, characterized by transabdominal migration. The hormonal control of the gubernacular swelling reaction remains controversial, with the persistent müllerian duct syndrome, as an experiment of nature, strongly supporting a role for MIS. The oestrogen-treated mouse also points to a role for MIS. Recent preliminary studies with the mouse gubernaculum in organ culture suggest MIS has a direct effect (Attah *et al.*, unpublished observations). Failure of anti-MIS antibodies to prevent gubernacular enlargement in the rabbit fetus, as well as failure of purified bovine MIS to stimulate gubernacular fibroblasts in tissue culture remain as significant negative results. Now that human recombinant MIS is becoming more widely available this controversy should be resolved by further direct experimentation.

References

1. Hutson JM. A biphasic model for the hormonal control of testicular descent. *Lancet* 1985; **ii:** 419–21.
2. Hutson JM, Donahoe PK. The hormonal control of testicular descent. *Endocr Rev* 1986; **7:** 270–83.
3. Wensing CJG, Colenbrander B, Van Straaten HWM. Normal and abnormal testicular descent in some mammals. In: Hafez ESE, ed. *Clinics in Andrology: Descended and Cryptorchid Testis*, The Hague, Martinus, Nijhoff, 1980: Vol 3, pp. 125–37.
4. Rajfer J. Hormonal regulation of testicular descent. *Eur J Pediatr* 1987; **146 (Suppl. 2):** S6–S7.

5. Rajfer J, Walsh PC. Hormonal regulation of testicular descent: experimental and clinical observations. *J Urol* 1977; **118:** 985–90.
6. Green RR, Burrill MW, Ivy AC. Experimental intersexuality. The effects of estrogens on the antenatal sexual development of the rat. *Am J Anat* 1940; **67:** 305–45.
7. Jean C. Croissance et structure des testicules cryptorchides chez les souris nees de mères traitées à l'oestradiol pendant à la gestation. *Ann Endocrinol* 1973; **34:** 669-87.
8. Hadziselimovic F, Herzog B, Kruslin E. Estrogen-induced cryptorchidism in animals. *Clin Androl* 1980; **3:** 166–74.
9. Newbold RR, Suzuki Y, McLachlan JA (1984). Müllerian duct maintenance in heterotypic organ culture after *in vivo* exposure to diethylstilbestrol. *Endocrinology* 1984; **115:** 1863–8.
10. Hutson JM. Exogenous oestrogens prevent transabdominal testicular descent in mice with complete androgen resistance (testicular feminisation). *Pediatr Surg Int* 1987; **2:** 242–6.
11. Habenicht UF, Neumann F (1983). Hormonal regulation of testicular descent. *Adv Anat Embryol Cell Biol* 1983; **81:** 1–54.
12. Wensing CJG, Colenbrander B. Normal and abnormal testicular descent. In: Clarke JR, ed. *Oxford Reviews of Reproductive Biology*. Oxford: Clarendon Press, 1986: Vol. 8, pp. 129–30.
13. Wensing CJG. Testicular descent in some domestic mammals. II. The nature of the gubernacular change during the process of testicular descent in the pig. *Proc Kon Ned Akad Wetensch Ser C* 1973; **76:** 190–5.
14. Wensing CJG. Testicular descent in the rat and a comparison of this process in the rat with that in the pig. *Anat Rec* 1986; **214:** 154–60.
15. Wells LJ. Descent of the testis: anatomical and hormonal considerations. *Surgery* 1943; **14:** 436–72.
16. Lewis LG. Cryptorchidism. *J Urol* 1948; **60:** 345–56.
17. Backhouse KM, Butler H. The gubernaculum testis of the pig (sus scropha). *J Anat* 1960; **94:** 107–21.
18. Backhouse KM. Embryology of testicular descent and maldescent. *Urol Clin N Am* 1982; **9:** 315–25.
19. Heyns CF, Human HJ, de Klerk DP. Hyperplasia and hypertrophy of the gubernaculum during testicular descent in the fetus. *J Urol* 1986; **135:** 1043–7.
20. Baumans V, Dijkstra G, Wensing CJG. The effect of orchidectomy on gubernaculum outgrowth and regression in the dog. *Int J Androl* 1982; **5:** 387–400.
21. Baumans V, Dijkstra G, Wensing CJG (1983). The role of a non-androgenic testicular factor in the process of testicular descent in the dog. *Int J Androl* 1983; **6:** 541–52.
22. Wensing CJG, Colenbrander B, Bosma AA. Testicular feminisation syndrome and gubernacular development in a pig. *Proc Kon Ned Akad Wetensch Ser C* 1975; **78:** 402–5.
23. Fentener van Vlissingen JM, Colenbrander B, Verbruggen A, Wensing CJG (1984). Testicular feminized males (TFM) in *Nyctereutes procyonoides* (Raccoon dog). In *Recent Progress in Cellular Endocrinology of the Testis*, INSERM Symposium, No 123, Amsterdam: Elsevier, 1984, pp. 335–40.
24. Hutson JM. Testicular feminization: a model for testicular descent in mice and men. *J Pediatr Surg* 1986; **21:** 195–8.
25. Wensing CJG, Colenbrander B. The process of normal and abnormal testicular descent. In: Bierich JR, Rager K, Ranke MB, eds. *Maldescensus Testis*. Baltimore: Urban and Schwarzenberg, 1977: pp. 193–7.
26. Husmann DD, McPhaul MJ. Localization of the androgen receptor in the developing rat gubernaculum. *Endocrinology* 1991; **128:** 383–7.

27. Heyns CF, Pape VC. Presence of a low capacity androgen receptor in the gubernaculum of the pig fetus. *J Urol* 1991; **145:** 161–7.
28. Spencer JR, Torrado T, Sanchez RS, Vaughan ED, Imperato-McGinley J. Effects of flutamide and finasteride on rat testicular descent. *Endocrinology* 1991; **129:** 741–8.
29. Hadziselimovic F, Herzog B, Kruslin E. Morphological background of oestrogen-induced cryptorchidism. *Pediatr Adolesc Endocrinol* 1979; **6:** 79–87.
30. Hadziselimovic F. Embryology of testicular descent and maldescent. In: Hadziselimovic F, ed. *Cryptorchidism*, Berlin: Springer-Verlag, 1983: pp. 11–34.
31. Hutson JM, Watts LM, Montalto J, Greco S. Both gonadotropin and testosterone fail to reverse estrogen-induced cryptorchidism in fetal mice: further evidence for non-androgenic control of testicular descent in the fetus. *Pediatr Surg Int* 1990a; **5:** 13-18.
32. Hutson JM, Williams MPL, Fallat ME, Attah A. Testicular descent: new insights into its hormonal control. In: Milligan S, ed. *Oxford Reviews of Reproductive Biology*, Vol. 12, Oxford: Clarendon Press, 1990b: pp. 1–56.
33. Grocock CA, Charlton HM, Pike MC. Role of the fetal pituitary in cryptorchidism induced by exogenous maternal oestrogen during pregnancy in mice. *J Reprod Fertil* 1988; **83:** 295–300.
34. Josso N, Fekete C, Cachin O, Nezelof C, Rappaport R. Persistence of Müllerian ducts in male pseudohermaphroditism, and its relationship to cryptorchidism. *Clin Endocrinol* 1983; **19:** 247–58.
35. Luthra M, Hutson JM. Late gestation exogenous oestrogen inhibits testicular descent in fetal mice despite Müllerian duct regression. *Pediatr Surg Int* 1990; **4:** 260–4.
36. Raynaud A. Inhibition, sous l'effet d'une hormone oestrogene, du developpement du gubernaculum du foetus male de souris. *Comp Rend Seanc Acad Sci* 1958; **246:** 176–9.
37. Josso N, Picard J-Y. Anti-Müllerian hormone. *Physiol Rev* 1986; **66:** 1038–90.
38. Hutson JM, Ikawa H, Donahoe PK. Estrogen inhibition of Müllerian inhibiting substance in the chick embryo. *J Pediatr Surg* 1982; **17:** 953–9.
39. Doi O, Hutson JM. Pretreatment of chick embryos with estrogen *in ovo* prevents Müllerian duct regression in organ culture. *Endocrinology* 1988; **122:** 2888–91.
40. Brook CGD. Persistent Müllerian duct syndrome. *Pediatr Adol Endoc* 1981; **8:** 100–4.
41. Sloan WR, Walsh PC. Familial persistent Müllerian duct syndrome. *J Urol* 1976; **115:** 459–61.
42. Beheshti M, Churchill BM, Hardy BE, Bailey JD, Weksberg R, Rogan GF. Familial persistent Müllerian duct syndrome. *J Urol* 1984; **131:** 968–9.
43. Josso N, Tran D. Biochemical aspects of prenatal testicular development: relationship to testicular descent. *Pediatr Androl Endocrinol 1979;* **6:** 37–46.
44. Hutson JM, Chow CW, Ng WD. Persistent Müllerian duct syndrome with transverse testicular ectopia. An experiment of nature with clues for understanding testicular descent. *Pediatr Surg Int* 1987; **2:** 191–4.
45. Scott JES. The Hutson hypothesis. *Br J Urol* 1987; **60:** 74–6.
46. Picard JY, Tran D, Vigier B, Josso N (1983). Maintien des canaux de Müller chez le lapin male par immunisation passive contre l'hormone anti-müllerienne pendant la vie foetale. *Comp Rend Seanc Acad Sci Ser III* 1983; **297:** 567–70.
47. Fentener van Vlissingen JM, van Zoelen EJJ, Ersem PJF, Wensing CJG. *In vitro* model of the first phase of testicular descent: identification of a low-molecular weight factor from fetal testis involved in proliferation of gubernaculum testis cells and distinct from specified polypeptide growth factors and fetal gonadal hormones. *Endocrinology* 1988; **123:** 2868–77.

3

Inguinoscrotal descent of the testis

3.1 Migration of the gubernaculum

The inguinoscrotal phase of testicular descent begins at 26 weeks in the human fetus.[1,2] Between weeks 26 and 28 of gestation, the testis descends rapidly through the inguinal canal, and then moves more slowly towards the scrotum, reaching it at 35 to 40 weeks.[2] In the human, migration of the gubernaculum and the testis occur simultaneously (Figures 3.1 and 3.2) while in rodents, migration of the gubernaculum preceeds testicular descent.[3,4] In rats, the gubernaculum migrates from the inguinal region to the scrotum between three and ten days postnatally, and in the mouse this occurs by about one week.[5] Migration of the rodent testis is delayed until the onset of pubertal hormone stimulation, which in the mouse occurs at about 2 weeks and in the rat at 3–4 weeks. Prior to the inguinoscrotal phase of migration, the gubernaculum ends at the abdominal wall, as shown a century ago by Cleland[5] and more recently by Fallat *et al.*,[6] and demonstrated in Figure 3.1

The processus vaginalis initially forms as a small evagination of the peritoneum into the gubernacular mesenchyme at the site of the future internal inguinal ring (Figure 3.3).[1] This peritoneal diverticulum later elongates within the gubernaculum to form an annular cavity, dividing the gubernaculum into a central mesenchymal column and an outer parietal layer (Figure 3.4) Following complete descent of the testis, the central gubernacular column involutes by dissolution of the extra-cellular matrix. The residual tissue of the column forms the fibrous attachment of the testis to the scrotum (Figure 3.5).

The cremaster muscle develops within the outer parietal layer of the gubernaculum, forming a bilaminar sac in rodents, and a strip of muscle

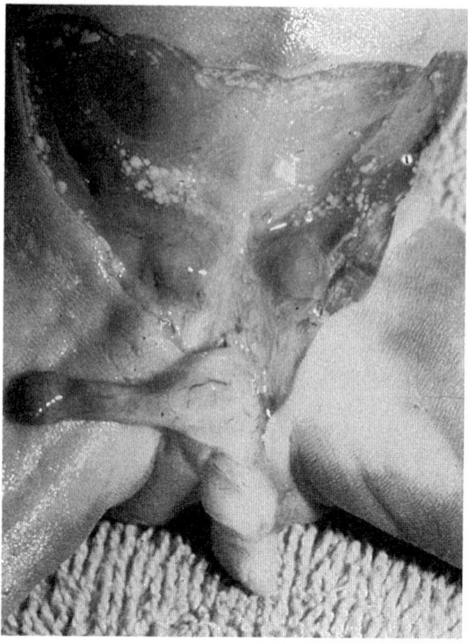

Figure 3.1 Dissection of 30-week human fetus showing gubernaculum emerging from the external ring. (Reproduced with permission of the publisher from Reference 2.)

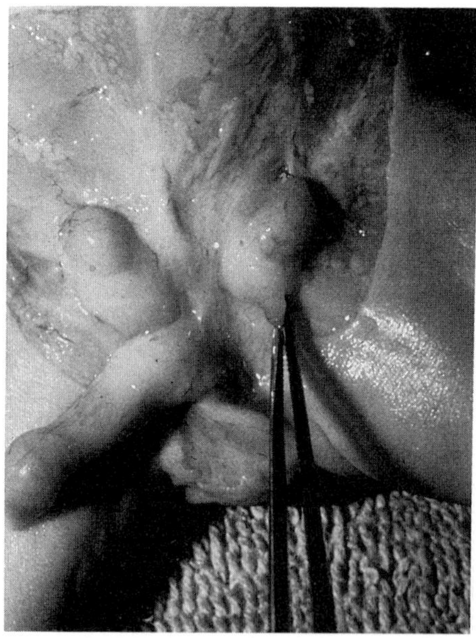

Figure 3.2 Dissection of 32-week human fetus showing the gubernaculum and testis migrating across the pubic region towards the scrotum. A pair of forceps holds up the free caudal end of the gubernaculum. (Reproduced with permission of the publisher from Reference 2.)

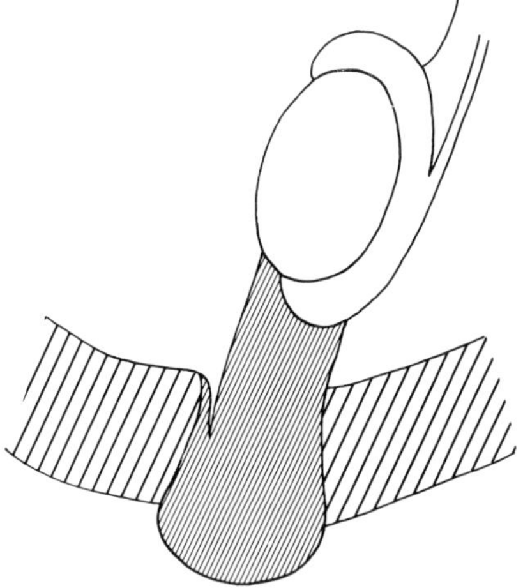

Figure 3.3 The gubernaculum with its developing processus vaginalis prior to inguinoscrotal descent.

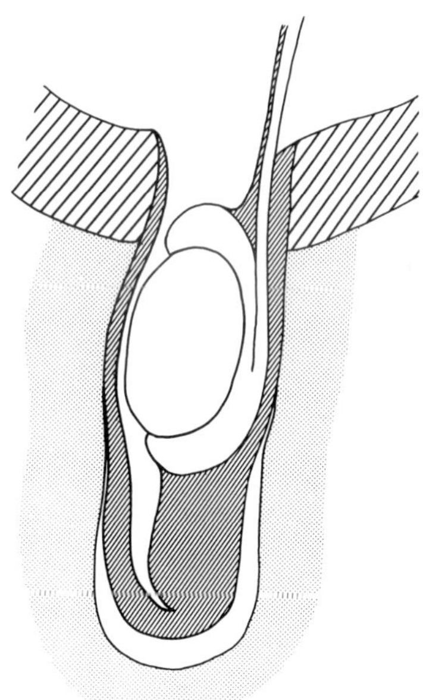

Figure 3.4 The gubernaculum during inguino-scrotal descent showing the processus vaginalis elongating within the mesenchyme to create a central column and an outer parietal layer. The caudal end is not attached to the surrounding inguinal mesenchyme.

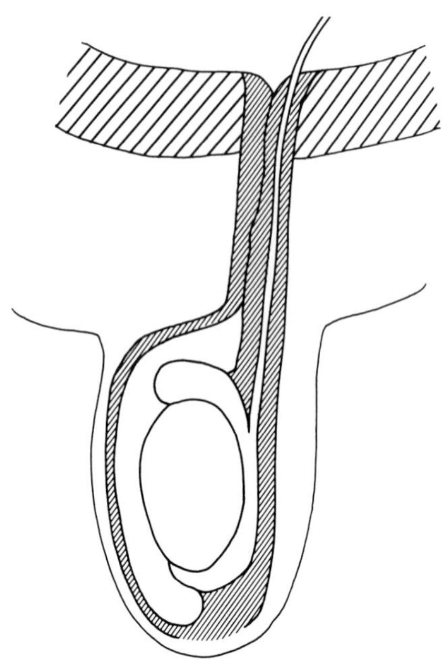

Figure 3.5 The gubernaculum after descent and involution of the central column.

in ungulates and primates.[7] The attachment of the cremaster muscle to the inguinal abdominal wall varies from species to species,[4] and is supplied by its own nerve: the genital branch of the genitofemoral nerve.[8,9]

During gubernacular migration, the gubernaculum in the human is ovoid or spherical, while in the rodent it is conical. Careful dissection of the distal end of the gubernaculum in humans (Figure 3.2),[2] pigs[1] and rodents[6] shows that the lower end of the gubernaculum is free and unattached to the adjacent mesenchyme. This has been used as evidence against the concept of the gubernaculum pulling the testis down to the scrotum, since it is not anchored inferiorly.[1,2] An alternative, however, is that the gubernaculum is migrating towards the scrotum by clearing the space ahead of it by enzymatic digestion (Figure 3.6). A potentially fruitful area of research, therefore, will be histochemical analysis of this region looking for evidence of enzymatic activity.

3.2 Intra-abdominal pressure

The force required to produce elongation of the processus vaginalis may be intra-abdominal pressure: this has long been assumed to push the testis down the inguinal canal[10] Recent studies on rats also suggest an important

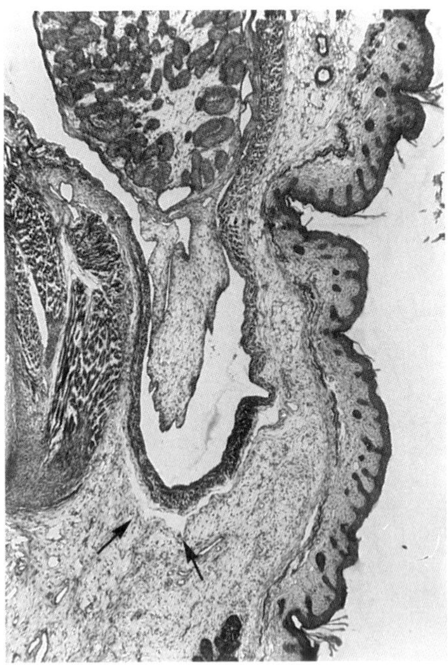

Figure 3.6 A photomicrograph of the gubernaculum during inguino-scrotal descent in a rat, showing the clear space just ahead of the leading edge of the gubernaculum (arrows).

role for abdominal pressure (Figure 3.7).[11–14] This possibility is supported by the fact that male human infants with severe abdominal wall defects, where abdominal pressure is lower than normal, have a high incidence of undescended testes[15] (see Chapter 4).

3.3 The role of testosterone

Experimental studies in rodents have suggested an important role for androgens in inguinoscrotal descent.[16–18] For example, androgen treatment or gonadotrophin treatment in immature rats causes premature testicular descent.[16] This effect of androgen treatment in prepubertal animals may be misleading, however, since Backhouse[1] has suggested that the important anatomical developments have been completed shortly after birth in the rodent and that subsequent hormonal treatment essentially is stimulating precocious puberty. Nevertheless, the failure of gubernacular migration and descent of the testis beyond the inguinal region in animals with testicular feminization demonstrates conclusively that androgens are crucial for this phase of descent. Even in the human with complete androgen resistance the testis never descends beyond the

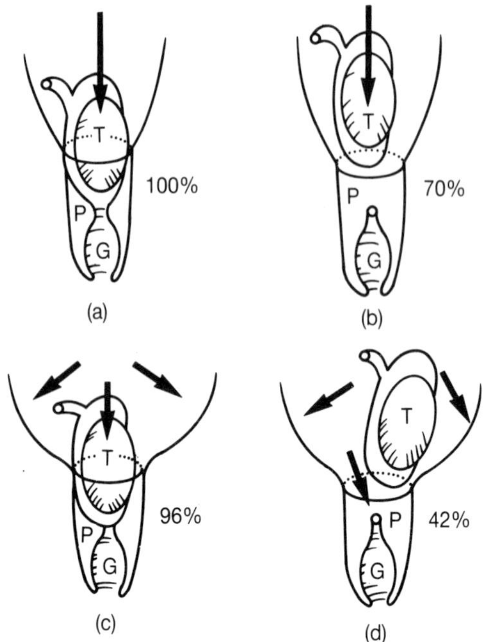

Figure 3.7 Schema showing the effect of either transection of the gubernaculum or creation of an abdominal wall defect on testicular descent in rats. G = Gubernaculum; P = pubis; T = testes. (a) Control rats; (b) transected gubernaculum;(c) surgically-created abdominal wall defect; (d) abdominal wall defect plus transected gubernaculum. Testicular descent is inhibited most in (d).

inguinal region (see Figure 2.3b, page 22).[19] In the rare genetic disorders of hypothalamic dysfunction inguinoscrotal descent is deficient.[20,21]

All these studies confirm that androgens are important for inguinoscrotal descent and gubernacular migration. The gubernaculum was believed by many workers to be the target organ for androgens, but this has not been proven by the presence of androgen receptors within the gubernaculum.[17] Oprins *et al.*[22] claimed to have found specific androgen receptors in cultured gubernacular fibroblasts derived from the fetal pig, but the total concentration of receptor in the pig gubernaculum was significantly less than in typical target tissues for androgen.[23] George and Peterson[24] found that the total amount of specific androgen which binds in the neonatal rat gubernaculum was one-fifth the amount measurable in the urogenital sinus. Recently, Heyns and Pape[25] looked carefully at the androgen binding in the fetal pig gubernaculum, and found both the receptor binding affinity and capacity was significantly lower than that of typical androgenic target tissues, such as the prostate and urethra. Androgen receptors have been localized within the mesenchymal core of the fetal rat gubernaculum, but the level of their expression decreases during the inguino-scrotal phase.[26]

The anti-androgen, flutamide, causes inhibition of inguino-scrotal descent in rats, but only when the compound is given between 12 and 18 days of gestation, and not when inguino-scrotal descent actually occurs, at 3–28 days after birth.[27] Although administration of oestrogens postnatally can prevent testicular descent,[28] postnatal anti-androgens had no effect at all. This apparently paradoxical response to anti-androgens can be understood once the role of the genitofemoral nerve is appreciated, as described below. Oestrogen administration is believed to inhibit pubertal development of the testis, such that it remains very small and never descends. By contrast, the migration of the gubernaculum to the scrotum postnatally is largely unaffected by oestrogen treatment (Griffiths and Hutson, unpublished observations). Since the normal migration of the gubernaculum beyond the groin is absent in androgen-resistant mice (Griffiths and Hutson, unpublished observations), this process is definitely androgen-dependent, but cannot be inhibited by simultaneous androgen blockade.

3.4 The genitofemoral nerve hypothesis

In 1948 Lewis[29] attempted to show that cremasteric contraction was the active step in testicular descent. He reasoned that since the genitofemoral nerve supplied the cremaster muscle, transection of the nerve would paralyse the muscle and prevent descent. He transected the genitofemoral nerve in newborn rats and found that this did prevent testicular descent, apparently supporting his hypothesis for cremasteric contraction. Many workers were critical of his experiment and conclusions, however, because they believed that contraction of the cremaster would pull the testis up to the groin, rather than down to the scrotum.

We have repeated this experiment and likewise found that transection of the genitofemoral nerve prevents inguinoscrotal descent of the testis in the neonatal rat.[30] In rats where the genitofemoral nerve was divided successfully at birth (Table 3.1), the testis remained intra-abdominal on the ipsilateral side. The effect of nerve transection was greatest in the first 2 days after birth, and thereafter there was a diminished effect on gubernacular migration. After 4 days there was no effect at all. These studies suggest a crucial role for the genitofemoral nerve in gubernacular migration. At first, however, we were unable to explain why nerve transection caused the gubernaculum to lose its apparent sensitivity to hormone stimulation. The need for an intact nerve supply did not concur with other endocrinological systems, where target organs remain sensitive to their specific hormone despite complete denervation or even transplantation. To overcome this difficulty, we proposed the simple hypothesis that the testosterone may act primarily on the genitofemoral nerve in the central nervous system, rather than directly on the gubernaculum. The

Table 3.1 Effect of division of genitofemoral nerve on testicular descent

		Genitofemoral nerve divided			Genitofemoral nerve intact		
Rat No.	Age when killed (days)	Testicular position	Testicular weight(g)	Spermatogen	Testicular position	Testicular weight(g)	Spermatogen
1	114	Abdominal	0.63	Low	Scrotal	1.51	Normal
2	76	Abdominal	0.46	Low	Scrotal	1.48	Normal
3	62	Abdominal	0.11	Low	Scrotal	1.55	Normal
4	98	Abdominal	0.43	Low	Scrotal	1.75	Normal
5	37	Abdominal	0.14	Low	Scrotal	0.25	Normal
6	37	Abdominal	0.31	Low	Scrotal	0.31	Normal
7	31	Abdominal	0.13	Low	Scrotal	0.15	Normal
8	31	Abdominal	0.24	Low	Scrotal	0.26	Normal

Reproduced with permission from Reference 30.

genitofemoral nerve could then act as an effective 'second messenger' for androgenic stimulation of the gubernaculum (Figure 3.8).[31]

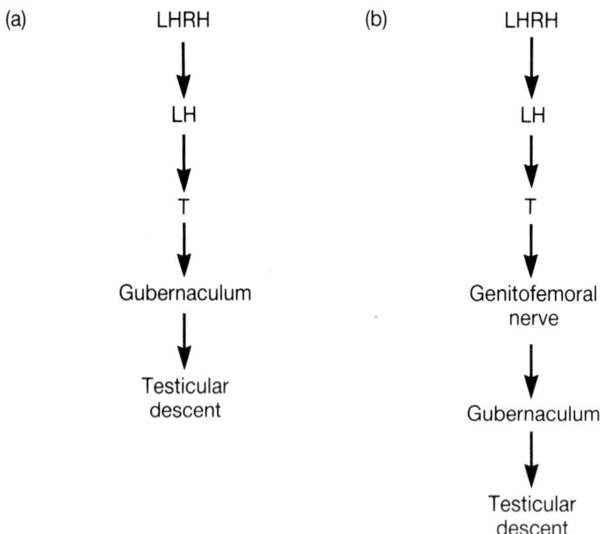

Figure 3.8 Schema showing hypothesis (A) that testosterone (T) acts directly on the gubernaculum to cause testicular descent, compared with hypothesis (B) that (T) acts indirectly on the gubernaculum via the genitofemoral nerve.

If the genitofemoral nerve was required for gubernacular migration, one would expect spinal cord abnormalities to be associated with undescended testes. This is in fact the case for children with spina bifida, particularly where the myelomeningocele is in the high lumbar region, the origin of the genitofemoral nerve (Figure 3.9).[32] A similar result can be obtained in the laboratory when the spinal cord of neonatal rats is transected: if this is performed in the low thoracic or high lumbar region, 75% of the testes were undescended (Table 3.2).[32]

Table 3.2 Effect of neonatal spinal cord transection on testicular descent in the rat

Level of Transection	Number of testes	Number (%) of undescended testes
Low thoracic/ high lumbar	4	3 (75)
Midlumbar	18	7 (39)
Lumbosacral	16	1 (6)

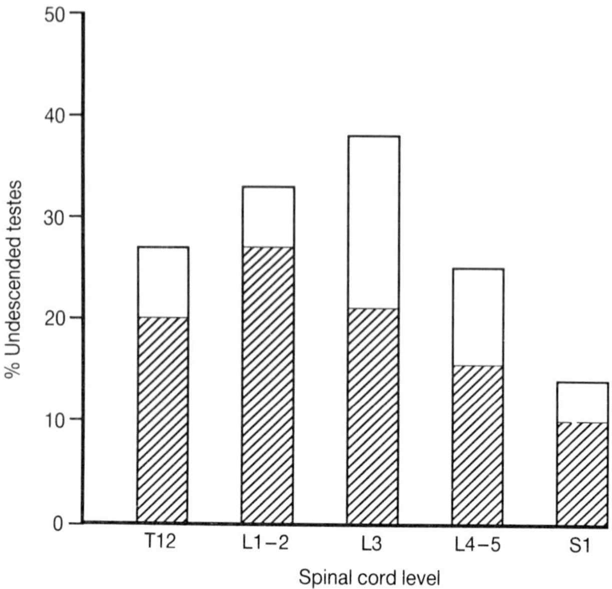

Figure 3.9 The percentage of undescended testes relative to the spinal level of paralysis in over 300 boys with spina bifida. Unilateral undescended testes are shown in open histograms and bilateral ones in cross-hatching.

3.5 Sexual dimorphism of genitofemoral nerve

For the genitofemoral nerve to be the mediator of androgen it would be necessary for it to be sexually dimorphic, i.e. it should be structurally modified by androgens in the male. This is indeed the case for the anterior spinal nucleus of the nerve in adult rats where the motor nucleus in the male contains approximately twice as many neurones as in the female. In addition, the cross-sectional area of the cell bodies in the male rat is greater than in the female.[33,34] We have repeated these studies in neonatal rats during the time of gubernacular migation and have demonstrated similar findings (Figure 3.10).[35] Moreover, we were able to identify a specific neuropeptide neurotransmitter within the cell bodies of the motor nucleus of the genitofemoral nerve which also was sexually dimorphic.[35] We assumed that if the genitofemoral nerve released a neurotransmitter as a second messenger for androgenic action on the gubernaculum, this messenger was likely to be a neuropeptide, that in other circumstances might function as a hormone. We tested a number of neuropeptide neurotransmitters with immunohistochemistry on the genitofemoral nucleus and identified that calcitonin gene-related peptide (CGRP) was found specifically within this nucleus. Approximately half the cells in the male and a quarter of the cells in the female were found

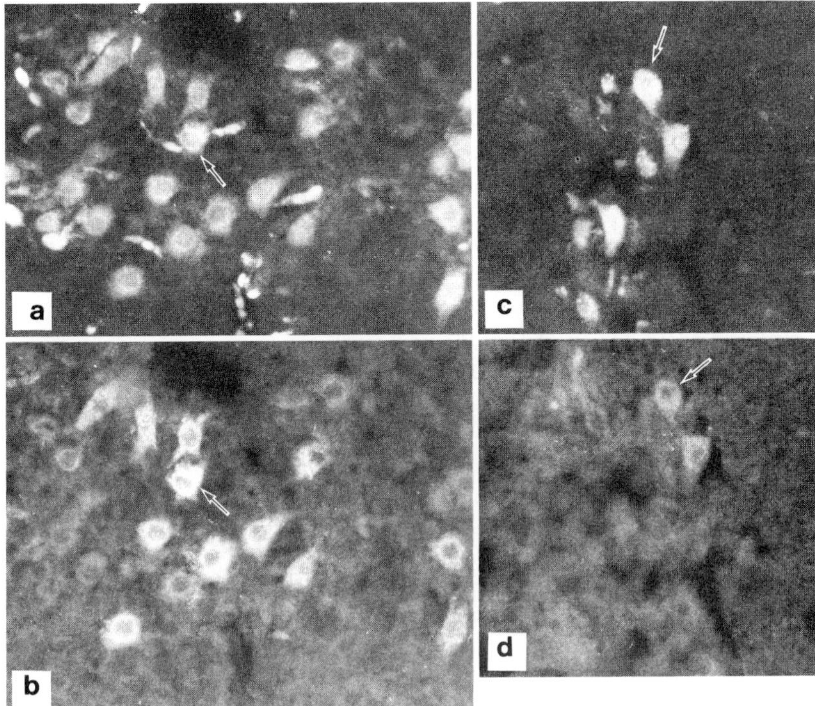

Figure 3.10 (a) Fluorescent dye (DAPI) labelling of the spinal nucleus of the genitofemoral nerve in a neonatal male rat (×240). The arrow marks the same cell in (a) and (b). (b) Immunohistochemical labelling of CGRP in the same section as (a) (×240). (c) Fluorescent labelling (DAPI) of the spinal nucleus in a neonatal female rat (×240). The arrow marks the same cell in (c) and (d). (d) Immunohistochemistry for CGRP in the same section as (c) (×240). (Reproduced with permission of the publisher from Reference 35.)

to contain this neuropeptide on immunohistochemistry. The actual cell numbers containing this neurotransmitter in male rats were approximately five times that of female rats. Such a large degree of sexual dimorphism in the distribution of this neurotransmitter suggests that it might have a role in gubernacular development.

In a related study we found that the genitofemoral nerve had branches containing CGRP which supplied the scrotal region ahead of the migrating gubernaculum (Figure 3.11).[36] The unique position of the genitofemoral nerve in the scrotal region, and its sexually dimorphic neurotransmitter CGRP, were consistent with our hypothesis that the nerve may release CGRP as a second messenger for androgenic control of the gubernaculum in its migration.

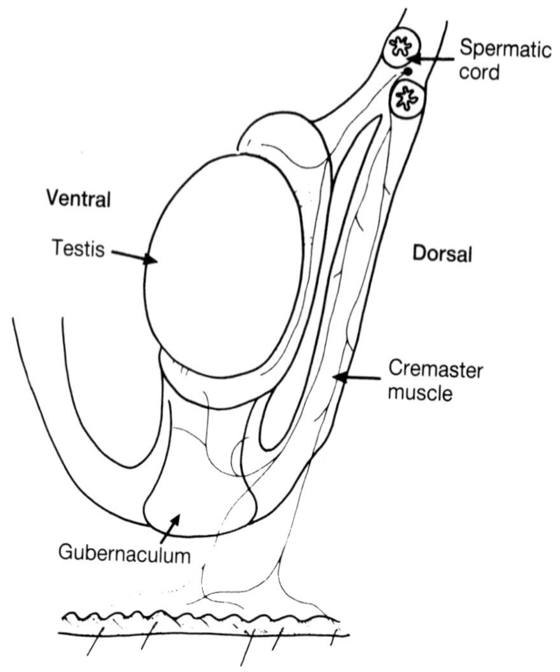

Figure 3.11 Schematic diagram of the course of the genitofemoral nerve to the scrotum. (Reproduced with permission of the publisher from Reference 36.)

3.6 The effect of CGRP

To determine the role, if any, of CGRP on the gubernaculum, we placed neonatal rat gubernacula in organ culture and added various concentrations of CGRP. To our great surprise CGRP induced rhythmic contractions of the gubernacular cremaster muscle at rates of up to 250 contractions per minute (Figure 3.12).[37] This remarkable observation has changed totally our view of the gubernaculum. Prior to this observation we had always imagined that the gubernaculum was relatively inert mesenchyme. Now we appreciate that the gubernaculum is an actively contractile and motile structure.

Similar studies have been performed using the neonatal mouse gubernaculum in organ culture. About half the gubernacula placed in culture show endogenous contraction, and this increases in a dose-responsive manner when exogenous CGRP is added to the medium (Momose and Hutson, unpublished observations). When a synthetic antagonist of CGRP is added to the culture system, contractions can be inhibited in a dose-responsive way (CGRP8-37 is an analogue of CGRP that binds to the receptor but has no function). Furthermore, the neonatal TFM gubernaculum, removed from an animal with lack of the normal

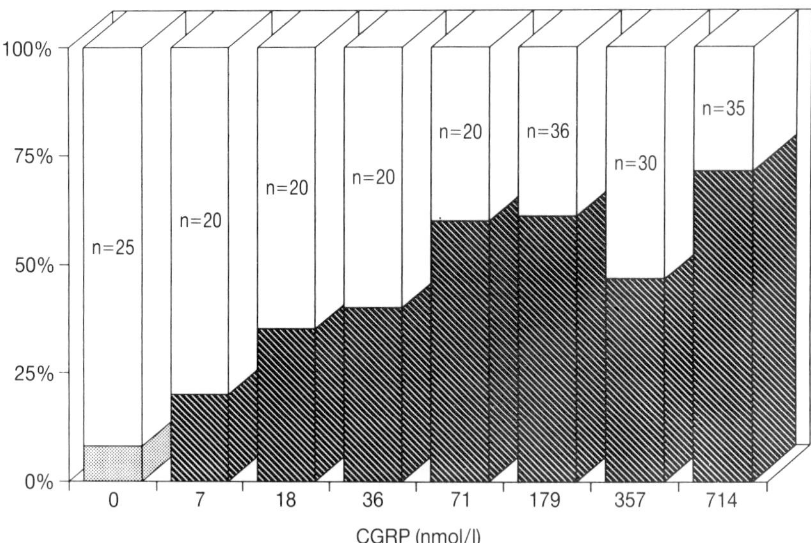

Figure 3.12 Number of contractile gubernacula at different concentrations of CGRP (n = 206), ⧅ fast contractions; ▒ slow contractions; □ non-contractile. The number on each column indicates the number of gubernacula. (Reproduced with permission of the publisher from Reference 37.)

masculinization of the genitofemoral nerve,[35] shows no endogenous contraction at all; when GCRP is added to the medium, the gubernacula respond with greatly enhanced contractions, consistent with hypersensitivity to CGRP (Momose and Hutson, unpublished observations).

Having observed rhythmic contraction of the gubernaculum in organ culture we looked at the gubernaculum *in situ* in neonatal rats under anaesthesia. Upon excision of the inguinoscrotal skin the gubernaculum is revealed to be a conical structure emerging from the inguinal canal. The caudal end of the gubernaculum is not attached, and this leading edge can twitch and is contractile. When the abdominal pressure is increased by manual compression, increasing the pressure within the processus vaginalis, the contractility of the gubernaculum becomes more vigorous.[37] The appearance of the gubernaculum is reminiscent of a windsock on a windy day.

Confirmation that CGRP has specific effects on the gubernaculum and direct involvement in testicular descent has been provided by the demonstration of specific binding sites for CGRP by autoradiography of neonatal rat gubernacula.[38]

In a related experiment, injection into neonatal mice of CGRP 8-37, an antagonist of CGRP (where the first seven amino acids of the peptide that are responsible for biological activity have been removed), caused a delay in testicular descent – from the normal 2 weeks, to 4 weeks, postnatally.[39]

3.7 Conclusion

Our work on the inguinoscrotal migration phase of the gubernaculum and testis has suggested an important role for the genitofemoral nerve. In addition, recent results suggest that neurotransmitters released from the genitofemoral nerve, such as CGRP, may mediate the action of androgens in a way analogous to a 'second messenger' (Figure 3.13). Other – as yet unknown – transmitters may be identified. It is not known whether all the functions controlled by androgen in this phase (such as gubernacular migration, processus vaginalis growth, cremaster development, and dissolution of the extra-cellular matrix) are done so via the genitofemoral nerve, or whether only the migration of the gubernaculum is controlled by the nerve. The intrinsic development of the gubernaculum, particularly the growth of the processus vaginalis and development of the cremaster, may be controlled directly by androgen receptors within the mesenchymal core. The exact role of the genitofemoral nerve remains to be fully defined. Research into this area could lead to new ways of treating undescended testis, since injection of the appropriate neurotransmitter theoretically may induce gubernacular migration postnatally in the human.

The paradoxical effect of the anti-androgen, flutamide, we think is caused by the fact that 'masculinization' of the genitofemoral nerve, an

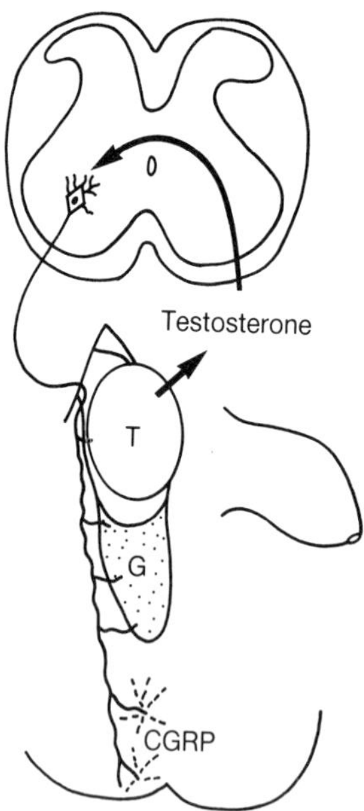

Figure 3.13 Schema showing how androgens may act via the genitofemoral nerve to modulate CGRP release as a 'second messenger' in the scrotum to induce gubernacular migration and testicular descent. (G = Gubernaculum; T = testis).

irreversible morphological change, probably occurs before gubernacular migration actually takes place, otherwise it could not provide the necessary directional signals. Other sexually dimorphic nuclei in the spinal cord are known to be differentiating during the last week of gestation in a rat,[40–42] so that this is the time that the inguino-scrotal phase of migration should be most sensitive to the androgen levels in the body. The maximum inhibitory effect of flutamide was between 15 and 17½ days of gestation, which is consistent with flutamide preventing inguino-scrotal descent indirectly by blocking masculinization of the genitofemoral nerve. Once the nerve has differentiated, the effect of androgens appears to be minimal.

References

1. Backhouse KM. Embryology of testicular descent and maldescent. *Urol Clin N Am* 1982; **9:** 315–25.
2. Heyns CF. The gubernaculum during testicular descent in the human fetus. *J Anat* 1987; **153:** 93–112.
3. Hadziselimovic F, Herzog B, Kruslin E. Morphological background of estrogen-induced cryptorchidism in the mouse. *Pediatr Adolesc Endocrinol* 1979; **6:** 79–87.
4. Wensing CJG. Testicular descent in the rat and a comparison of this process in the rat with that in the pig. *Anat Rec* 1986; **214:** 154–60.
5. Cleland J. *The Mechanism of the Gubernaculum Testis.* Prize thesis. Edinburgh: MacLachlan and Stewart, 1856: pp. 6–40.
6. Fallat ME, Williams MPL, Farmer PJ, Hutson JM. Histologic evaluation of inguinoscrotal migration of the gubernaculum in rodents during testicular descent and its relationship to the genitofemoral nerve. *Pediatr Surg Int* 1992 (In press).
7. Wensing CJG, Colenbrander B, Van Straaten HWM. Normal and abnormal testicular descent in some mammals. In: Hafez ESE, ed. *Clinics in Andrology: Descended and Cryptorchid Testis.* The Hague: Martinus Nijhoff, 1980: Vol. 3 pp. 125–37.
8. Hodson N. The nerves of the testis, epididymis and scrotum. In: Johnson AD, Gomes WR, Vandemark NL, eds. *The Testis.* New York: Academic Press; 1970: Vol.1, pp. 47–99.
9. Tayakkanonta K. The gubernaculum testis and its nerve supply. *Aust NZ J Surg* 1963; **33:** 61–7.
10. Hunter RH. The etiology of congenital inguinal hernia and abnormally placed testes. *Br J Surg* 1926; **15:** 125–30.
11. Frey HL, Peng S, Rajfer J. Synergy of abdominal pressure and androgens in testicular descent. *Biol Reprod* 1983; **29:** 1233–9.
12. Frey HL, Rajfer J. Role of the gubernaculum and intraabdominal pressure in the process of testicular descent. *J Urol* 1984; **131:** 574–9.
13. Quinlan DM, Gearheart JP, Jeffs RD. Abdominal wall defects and cryptorchidism: an animal model. *J Urol* 1988; **140:** 1141–4.
14. Attah AA, Hutson JM. The role of intraabdominal pressure in cryptorchidism 1992 (in press).
15. Kaplan LM, Martin AK, Kaplan GW, Farrer JH, Rajfer J. Associaiton between abdominal wall defects and cryptorchidism. *J Urol* 1986; **136:** 645–7.

16. Rajfer J, Walsh PC. Hormonal regulation of testicular descent: experimental and clinical observations. *J Urol* 1977; **118:** 985–90.
17. Rajfer J. Hormonal regulation of testicular descent. *Eur J Pediatr* 1987; **146 (Suppl. 2):** 56–7.
18. Johansen TEB. Therapeutic basis in cryptorchidism. A clinical and experimental study. *J Oslo City Hosp* 1988; **38:** 27–43.
19. Hutson JM. Testicular feminization: a model for testicular descent in mice and men. *J Pediatr Surg* 1986; **21:** 195–8.
20. Bardin CW, Ross GT, Rifkind AB, Cargille CM, Lipsett MB. Studies of the pituitary-Leydig cell axis in young men with hypogonadotropic hypogonadism and hyposmia: comparison with normal men, prepubertal boys, and hypopituitary patients. *J Clin Invest* 1969; **48:** 2046–56.
21. Cattanach BM, Idden CA, Charlton HM, Chiappa SA, Fink G. Gonadotrophin-releasing hormone deficiency in a mutant mouse with hypogonadism. *Nature* 1977; **269:** 338–40.
22. Oprins AC, Fentener van Vlissingen JM, Blankenstein MA. Testicular descent: androgen receptors in cultured porcine gubernaculum cells. *J Steroid Biochem* 1988; **31:** 387–91.
23. Heyns CF, Pape VC, De Klerk DP. Demonstration of a cytosolic androgen receptor in the gubernaculum of the pig fetus. *J Urol* 1988; **139:** 236A.
24. George FW, Peterson KG. Partial characterization of the androgen receptor of the newborn rat gubernaculum. *Biol Reprod* 1988; **39:** 536–9.
25. Heyns CF, Pape VC. Presence of a low capacity androgen receptor in the gubernaculum of the pig fetus. *J Urol* 1991; **145:** 161–7.
26. Husmann DA, McPhaul MJ. Localization of the androgen receptor in the developing rat gubernaculum. *Endocrinology* 1991; **128:** 383–7.
27. Spencer JR, Torrado T, Sanchez RS, Vaughan ED. Imperato-McGinlay J. Effects of flutamide and finasteride on rat testicular descent. *Endocrinology* 1991; **129:** 741–8.
28. Kogan BA, Gupta R, Juenemann KP. Fertility in cryptorchidism: further development of an experimental model. *J Urol* 1987; **137:** 128–31.
29. Lewis LG. Cryptorchidism. *J Urol* 1948; **60:** 345–6.
30. Beasley SW, Hutson JM. Effect of division of the genitofemoral nerve on testicular descent in the rat. *Aust NZ J Surg* 1987; **57:** 49–51.
31. Hutson JM, Beasley SW. Annotation. The mechanisms of testicular descent. *Aust Paed J* 1987; **23:** 215–6.
32. Hutson JM, Beasley SW, Bryan AD. Cryptorchidism in spina bifida and spinal cord transection: a clue to the mechanism of transinguinal descent of the testis. *J Pediatr Surg* 1988; **23:** 275–7.
33. Kojima M, Sano Y. Sexual differences in the topographical distribution of serotonergic fibres in the anterior column of rat lumbar spinal cord. *Anat Embryol* 1984; **170:** 117–21.
34. Kojima M, Takeuchi Y, Kawata M, Sano Y. Motoneurons innervating the cremaster muscle of the rat are characteristically densely innervated by serotonergic fibres as revealed by combined immunohistochemistry and retrogade fluorescence DAPI-labelling. *Anat Embryol* 1983; **168:** 41–9.
35. Larkins SL, Hutson JM, Williams MPL. Localisation of calcitonin gene-related peptide immunoreactivity within the spinal nucleus of the genitofemoral nerve. *Pediatr Surg Int* 1991; **6:** 176–9.
36. Larkins SL, Hutson JM. Fluorescent anterograde labelling of the genitofemoral nerve shows that it supplies the scrotal region before migration of the gubernaculum. *Pediatr Surg Int* 1991; **6:** 167–71.
37. Park WH, Hutson JM. The gubernaculum shows rhythmic contractility and active movement during testicular descent. *J Pediatr Surg* 1991; **26:** 1–3.

38. Yamanaka J, Metcalfe SA, Hutson JM. Demonstration of calcitonin gene-related peptide receptors in the gubernaculum by computerized densitometry. *J Pediatr Surg* 1992 (In press).
39. Samarakkody UKS, Hutson JM. Intrascrotal CGRP 8-37 causes a delay in testicular descent in mice. *J Pediatr Surg* 1992 (In press).
40. Breedlove SM. Hormonal control of the anatomical specificity of motoneuron-to-muscle innervation in rats. *Science* 1985; **227:** 1357–9.
41. Breedlove SM, Arnold AP. Hormonal control of a developing neuromuscular system. I. Complete demasculinization of the male rat spinal nucleus of the bulbocavernosus using the anti-androgen flutamide. *J Neurosci* 1983a; **3:** 417–23.
42. Breedlove SM, Arnold A. Hormonal control of a developing neuromuscular system. II. Sensitive periods for the androgen-induced masculinization of the rat spinal nucleus of the bulbocavernosus. *J Neurosci* 1983b; **3:** 424–32.

4

Classification and causes of undescended testes in humans

4.1 Classification of undescended testes

For the purposes of description and evaluation of results it is necessary to classify testes according to their position (Figure 4.1a,b). It has to be recognized, however, that the testis is not an immobile or fixed structure with a single location; instead, it has a 'range of movement'.[1] This movement is a result of the cremasteric reflex and contraction of the dartos muscle, and is a normal finding in all prepubertal boys. Movement of the testis is possible by virtue of its position within the processus vaginalis, as is seen particularly in the superficial inguinal pouch testis (Figure 4.1a): its loose attachments via the mesorchium enable the testis to move anywhere within the processus vaginalis.

An undescended testis is one that cannot be manipulated to the bottom of the scrotum without undue tension on the spermatic cord (see Chapter 6). The corollary of this is that a descended testis is one that resides spontaneously in the lower scrotum, irrespective of its position at the time it is first located.

The various terms which are used to describe the location of a testis which cannot be made to reach the bottom of the scrotum are discussed below.

4.1.1 Intra-abdominal testis

The testis is located in the abdominal cavity, usually within a centimetre or two of the internal inguinal ring. The vas deferens and vessels supplying it reach it extraperitoneally via the mesorchium. Surgically, the testis can be located either by opening the peritoneum at the internal ring or by following the extraperitoneal course of the testicular vessels and vas deferens, the latter as it runs from the base of the bladder. Clinically, the

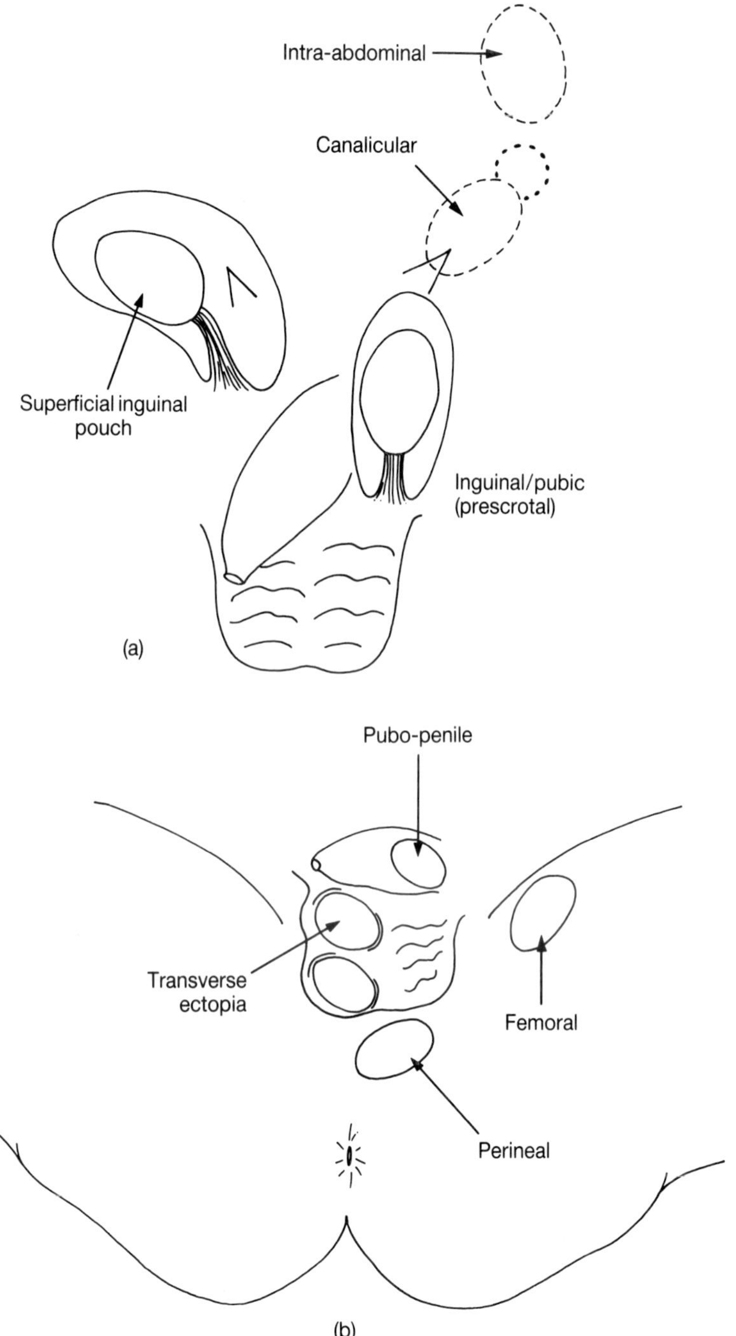

Figure 4.1 Range of positions which may be adopted by testes: (a) in the line of normal descent (including the superficial inguinal pouch); and (b) true ectopic sites, which are rare.

intra-abdominal testis is impalpable, but can be seen on laparoscopy (see Chapter 6).

4.1.2 Canalicular testis

A canalicular testis lies within the inguinal canal and is protected anteriorly by the aponeurosis of the external oblique muscle. The aponeurosis makes a canalicular testis difficult or impossible to palpate unless it can be coerced distally within its processus vaginalis through the external inguinal ring; in this situation it is described as being an 'emergent testis', referring to the fact that it has been made to emerge from the inguinal canal.[2]

4.1.3 Testis in superficial inguinal pouch

This is a somewhat confusing term which has been used to denote the processus vaginalis and its contained testis which has descended through the external ring to lie lateral or supero-lateral to the external inguinal ring (Figure 4.2). The testis has a longer spermatic cord than its intra-abdominal or canalicular counterpart and at orchidopexy requires relatively less mobilization of the cord to achieve a satisfactory position in the scrotum. These undescended testes are prevented from entering the scrotum by a fascial barrier which can be felt at operation. Because the

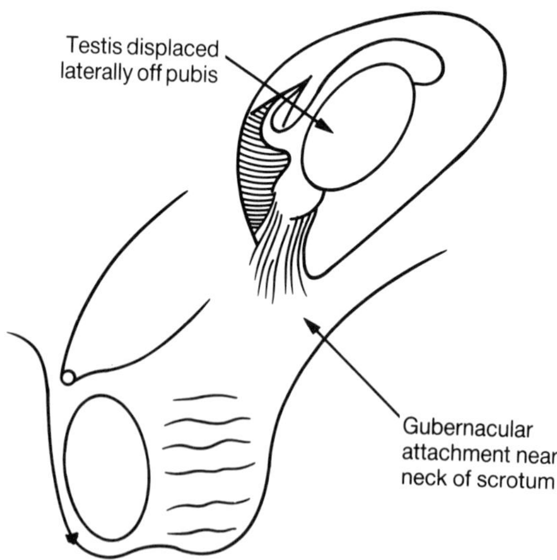

Figure 4.2 Testes in the 'superficial inguinal pouch'. Note that the gubernaculum is attached near the neck of the scrotum in most instances.

processus vaginalis does not extend into the scrotum, its contained testis cannot be manipulated into it. Browne[3] described the superficial inguinal pouch as lying anterior to the external oblique fascia just superior to the external inguinal ring. The roof of the pouch is formed by Scarpa's fascia and the posterior wall by the external oblique aponeurosis. Essentially, it is the space created by the processus vaginalis in the groin, and is limited by the extension of the external spermatic fascia from the external ring.

At times, an undescended testis in this position has been labeled as being 'ectopic'. For example, Jones[2] describes an 'arrested' testis as being small, ill-formed and relatively immobile with a short spermatic cord, lying usually near the pubic tubercle, while an 'ectopic' testis is normal in size with a good length of spermatic cord but which has diverged from its normal path during descent. It is not known, however, whether the superficial inguinal pouch is caused simply by passive deflection of the testis and processus vaginalis, or whether the gubernaculum actively migrated in the wrong direction and thereby failed to enter the neck of the scrotum.

4.1.4 The 'obstructed' testis

The 'obstructed' testis is a term not often used nowadays, but describes a testis palpable in the groin which cannot be made to enter the scrotum at all. The implication of the term is that there is transverse obstructing fascia at or above the neck of the scrotum which prevents the testis from descending beyond it.[3,4] Most authors would not distinguish these from testes in the superficial inguinal pouch. The testis itself is (initially) the same size as the contralateral descended testis and the spermatic cord is of adequate length, making transplantation into the scrotum easy. The barrier at the neck of the scrotum becomes obvious during surgical development of a path, down which the testis is to be brought. It is our belief that the main problem in the obstructed testis is failure of the processus vaginalis to extend caudally beyond the neck of the scrotum.

4.1.5 Ectopic testis

The truly ectopic testis has descended to a position other than the scrotum, and is not merely deflected or pushed laterally by the prominence of the pubis. Ectopic testes are described as being: femoral; perineal (Figure 4.3); pubopenile; or transverse (crossed) testicular ectopia.

The perineal testis is located in the perineum or high on the medial aspect of the thigh lateral to the entrance of the scrotum. Its significance is that unless specifically looked for, it can easily be missed at clinical examination and result in an erroneous conclusion of an impalpable or absent testis. The testis may be positioned a long way beyond the external ring and even the scrotum, and on some occasions lies not far from the

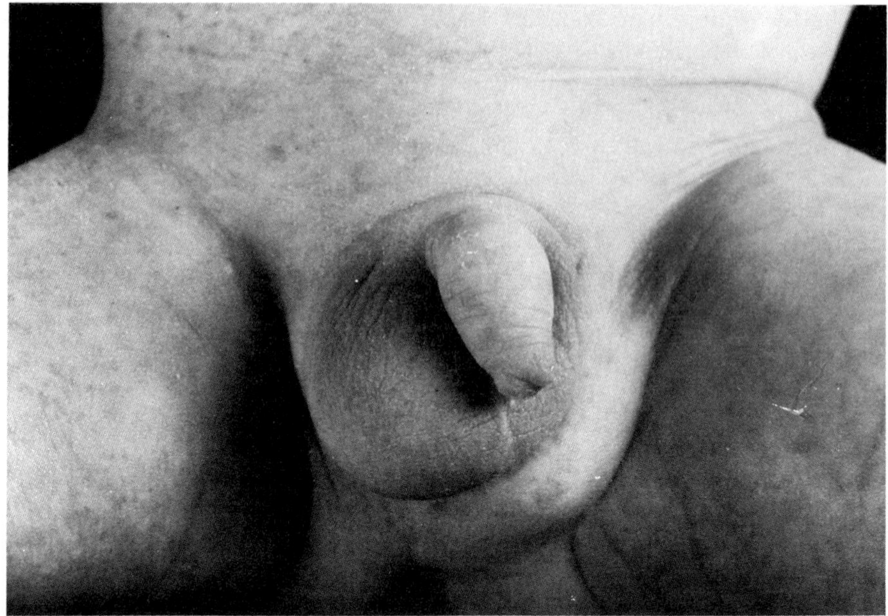

Figure 4.3 Perineal ectopic testis.

anus (Figure 4.3). Variants of ectopia include the so-called pubopenile testis, which lies at the base of the penis in a more medial position than the normal line of descent; and the crural or femoral testis, which is more obviously in the upper thigh. These ectopic positions of the testes, although rare, must be looked for in any child in whom the location of the testis is not immediately apparent.

Transverse testicular ectopia

Transverse testicular ectopia (crossed testicular ectopia) is an extremely rare but well recognised entity in which the clinical findings are those of a hernia on one side and an impalpable testis on the other.[5] The testis on the side of the hernia is normally found fully descended in the scrotum. The characteristic features of true descended crossed ectopia of the testis are: (i) two testes found on one side with no testis on the other side; (ii) the testes identical in size and appearance and each has its own epididymis, vas deferens and testicular vessels; (iii) an associated hernia on the side of the two testes with no hernia on the contralateral side.[6]

In about 20% of reports, crossed testicular ectopia has been described in association with persistence of müllerian structures.[7] Until recently, it has been unclear whether these cases should be included with those of simple crossed testicular ectopia, where the gubernaculum is disrupted or accidentally attached to the opposite inguinal region; or whether they constitute a separate condition which is part of a generalized genetic or endocrine abnormality.[6,8] A clue to its cause has been provided by recognition of the frequency in which transverse ectopia occurs in patients with persistent müllerian ducts, suggesting that müllerian duct retention is an important factor in its aetiology.[9] Despite persistence of the müllerian ducts, there is absence of the female homologue of the gubernaculum, the round ligament, that normally tethers the uterus, fallopian tubes and ovaries, and prevents ovarian descent from occurring. Absence of the round ligament in persistent müllerian duct syndrome allows greater movement of the testes, and without these gubernacular structures, there is nothing to guide the testis into the correct inguinal canal (see Figure 2.8, page 28). The result is that the testis can herniate readily into the contralateral canal as an 'accidental' effect under the influence of abdominal pressure, a factor that is believed to be important during normal descent through the inguinal canal.[10,11]

4.1.6 The retractile testis

Retraction of the testis into the upper scrotum (or even higher) is a normal phenomenon for regulating the temperature of the testis in children, and is also a protective reflex. The cremasteric reflex which causes retraction can be invoked by cold temperature, anxiety, nervousness or local stimulation, particularly in the region of the cutaneous distribution of the genitofemoral nerve (Figure 4.4).

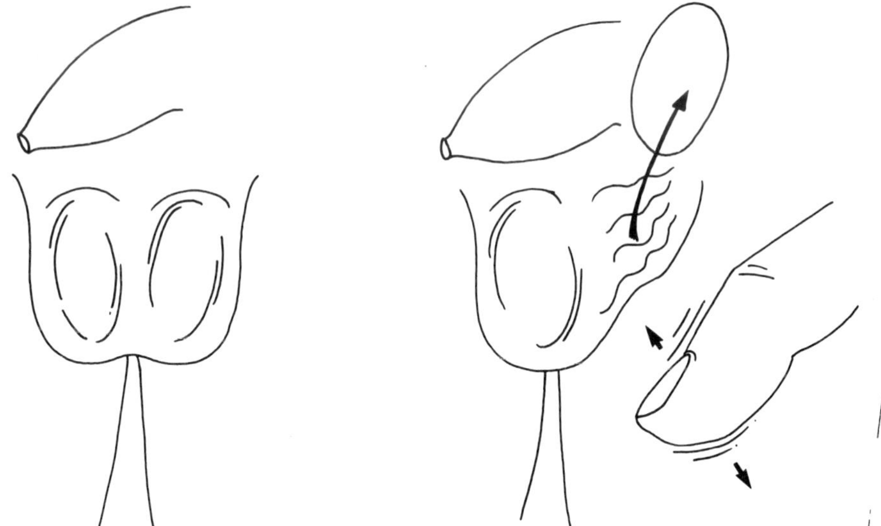

Figure 4.4 The retractile testis and reflex contraction of the cremaster muscle on stimulation of the inner side of the thigh (the cutaneous distribution of the genitofemoral nerve).

Retractility of the testis is normal in all prepubertal boys and is due to contraction of the cremaster muscle. This reflex can be stimulated by temperature changes or tactile stimulation of the inguino-scrotal region and inner side of the thigh, particularly in the distribution of the sensory branches of the genitofemoral nerve. Clinical experience suggests that the sensitivity of the reflex varies between children and with age.

At birth, the cremasteric reflex is either absent or extremely weak,[4] and between 3 and 9 years, is most pronounced. There appears to be an inverse relationship between serum testosterone levels and the activity of the cremasteric reflex (Figure 4.5), but the exact mechanism of this is yet to be clarified. The testis can appear to be out of the scrotum for so much of the time that differentiation from true non-descent may be difficult, and require periodic re-examination.

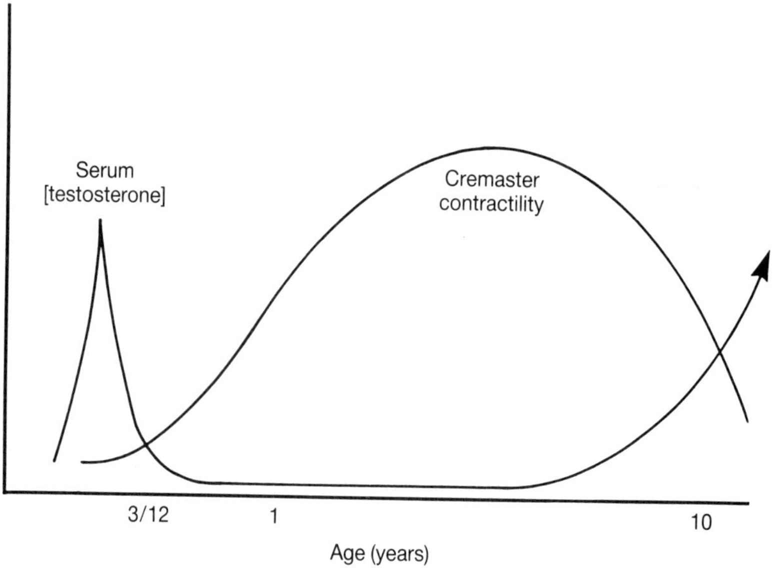

Figure 4.5 Relationship of the cremasteric reflex to age and the serum level of testosterone.

Farrington[12] found that, in boys aged 1 year, 20% of the testes were not visible in the scrotum on inspection, and by 4 years this figure had risen to 30%. Beyond 12 years, the testes were all located at the bottom of the scrotum. In all patients he studied, the testes could be manipulated into the lower scrotum at any age. Farrington concluded that the testis was most retractile at 5–6 years, after which age stimulation of the cremasteric reflex became less able to retract the testis out of the scrotum. At birth the cremasteric reflex is not present.

In a study of 100 boys with retractile testes who were followed up for 5 years, Wyllie[13] found that retraction continued throughout childhood, and stopped shortly before puberty. He emphasized that even experienced clinicians may have difficulty in distinguishing retractile from incompletely descended testes and concluded that, when dealing with a retractile testis, the assumption of a normal position in the scrotum was not absolutely certain, and periodic review at regular intervals was therefore mandatory. Furthermore, he made the comment that it is not adequate to say 'The testis was brought to the scrotum'. He identified the testis as having three possible positions in the scrotum: the normal position is low in the scrotum, i.e. 70–75 mm from the pubic tubercle (age-dependent); the high scrotal level is 50 mm from the pubic tubercle; and the mid-scrotal position is 60 mm. A retractile testis that can only reach the high scrotal position is of much greater concern than one which assumes a low scrotal position.

It should be noted that paediatric surgeons have not reached complete agreement as to exactly what constitutes a 'retractile' testis. Most clinicians would agree that the implication of a retractile testis is that it is a descended one, although careful follow-up is required and occasionally it may produce a surprise. Most believe that retractility reflects a normal physiological response to contraction of the cremaster muscle, and has a direct relationship to age.

4.1.7 The ascending testis

A newly described variant of the retractile testis is called the 'ascending' testis. In this situation the testis appears to be located within the scrotum in early infancy, but then as the boy grows, the testis appears to ascend back out of the scrotum, commonly leading to orchidopexy late in childhood. It had been postulated that the cause of this delayed ascent with growth is failure of the processus vaginalis to involute, which leads to failure of the spermatic cord to elongate in proportion to the growth of the boy.[14] Orchidopexy is commonly performed on such children between 8 and 11 years, when the abnormality is most marked and anxiety about subsequent fertility leads to consultation. In a review of boys coming to orchidopexy at the Royal Children's Hospital in Melbourne, where 350 orchidopexies are performed per year, a significant percentage underwent surgery between 8 and 11 years (Figure 4.6).[15]

The cause of the so-called ascending testis is not known, but it has been shown recently by the propective study performed at the John Radcliffe Hospital in Oxford that these children often have delayed descent of the testis in the first 1–3 months after birth (Figure 4.7). The Radcliffe study group found the testes of these boys were not located in the scrotum on the day of birth but descended into the scrotum within 12 weeks. However, by 1 year of age the testis had reascended out of the scrotum and became progressively higher with age.[16] These children appear to have an intermediate abnormality where the spermatic cord fails

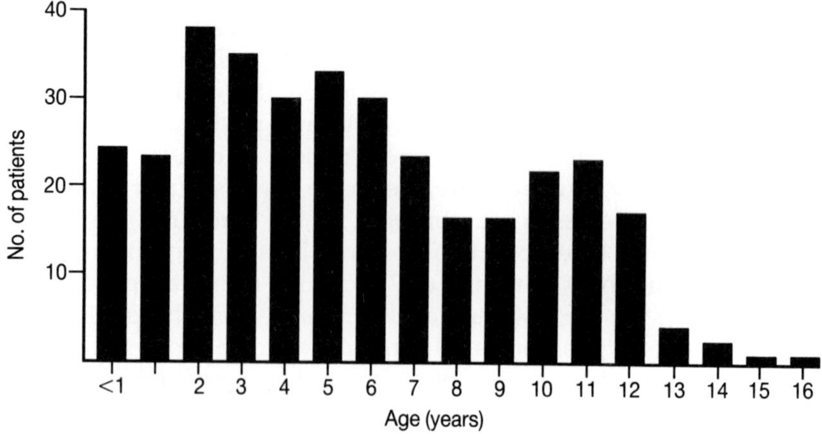

Figure 4.6 Age distribution in 350 boys admitted for orchidopexy at the Royal Children's Hospital, Melbourne. (Redrawn from Reference 15.)

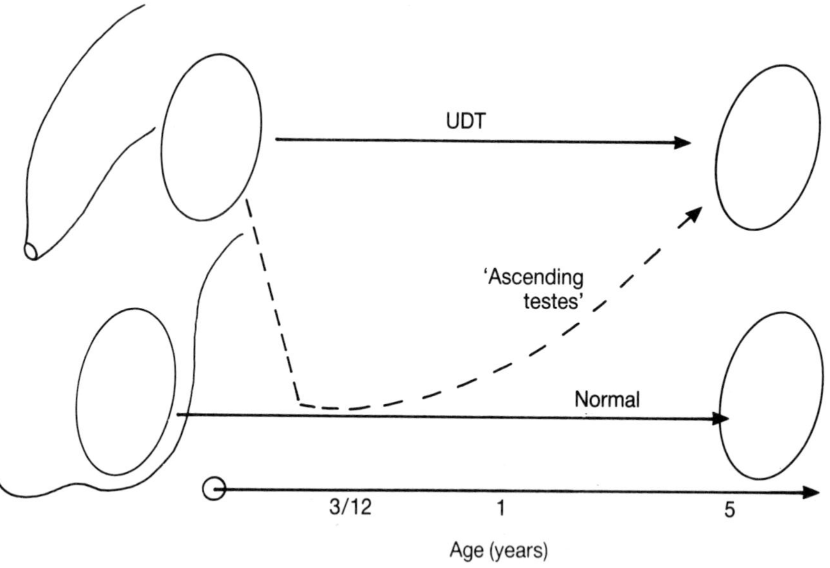

Figure 4.7 The relationship between the position of the testis at birth and at 5 years in descended (normal) testes, undescended and 'ascending' testes.

to elongate in proportion to body growth. This is in contrast to the normal situation where the spermatic cord elongates in proportion to body growth throughout childhood (Figure 4.8).

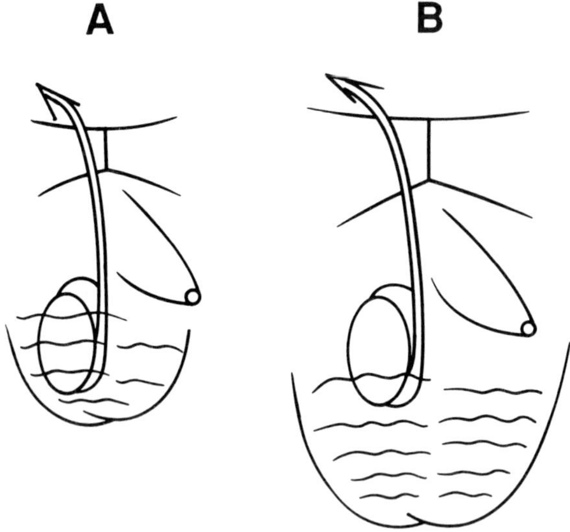

Figure 4.8 Failure of the spermatic cord to elongate in proportion to body growth may be a cause of ascending testes. (a) The testis descended in infancy assumes (b) a higher position later in childhood.

4.2 The incidence of undescended testis

The most widely quoted study investigating the incidence of undescended testes in the community is by Scorer[17] who surveyed more than 3500 male infants and found a 4.3% incidence of undescended testes. In full-term infants weighing more than 2500 g the incidence of cryptorchidism was 2.7% compared with 21% in premature infants (see Section 4.2.2). In an earlier study by Bishop[18] as many as 10% of newborn males were recorded as having cryptorchidism.

In an untreated population, the incidence of undescended testes decreases with age. Scorer found that 0.8% of 3612 boys examined at one year had an undescended testis. Other studies have suggested that 2% of males at age 1, and 1% at puberty, have cryptorchidism.[18,19] The massive review conducted by Campbell[20] involving 2.8 million United States Selective Service physical examinations reported an incidence of 0.44% in adult males, whereas Baumrucker[21] recorded the incidence in 10 000 consecutive inductees into the US army to be 0.75%. Failure to define accurately the level in the scrotum at which a testis is considered undescended makes it impossible to refine these figures further, other than to say that the incidence of non-descent was about 1% at 1 year of age. Beyond 1 year, it would seem that spontaneous descent of the testis is unlikely to occur,[22] and in fact probably does not occur beyond 3 months.

4.2.1 Increase in incidence of cryptorchidism

A recent review of orchidopexy rates in England and Wales suggested that the incidence of cryptorchidism may have doubled over the past 2 decades.[23] While it may be that the finding was a reflection of differences in the indications for orchidopexy and that some boys with retractile rather than cryptorchid testes are receiving surgery, there must be some concern that there is a genuine increase in the incidence of undescended testes. If this is so, there would be important implications in terms of fertility and the future incidence of testicular malignancy.[23] A subsequent study[16] has shown an apparent increase in incidence from 0.96% in 1960 to 1.58% in 1986. The 65% increase in incidence contrasted with the two-fold increase in the national orchidopexy rate. The proportion of boys undergoing orchidopexy was almost twice that of infants with an undescended testis at 3 months of age. Atwell[14] has suggested that this could be explained if it were established that in some cases cryptorchidism was acquired after birth by resorption of an occult inguinal hernia. The John Radcliffe Hospital Cryptorchidism Study Group[16] reported that 18 of 45 boys (40%) who testes descended after birth but before 3 months of age had an 'undescended' testis when followed up at 1 year. MacKellar *et al.*[24] made the observation that the increased frequency of operation bears a direct relationship to the lowering of the recommended age of operation, and it may reflect difficulty in excluding the child with a retractile testis from one with an incompletely descended testis.

4.2.2 Incidence of undescended testis in low-birthweight and low-gestation infants

There is a correlation between the degree of prematurity and the frequency of undescended testes.[25] In infants with a birthweight of less than 1500 g there is a 60–70% incidence of cryptorchidism.[26] This parallel with gestational age reflects the fact that the testes normally do not enter the scrotum until about 7 months' gestation.

Undescended testes are more common in low birthweight infants,[4] and it is presumed that this is mainly on account of their low gestational age. For example, in a study of testicular position at 18 months after term in 355 infants born under 1850 g, undescended testes were present in 29 out of 186 (16%) of those born under 1500 g ($p= 0.001$).[25] These data suggest that cryptorchidism is related strongly to birthweight. However, there is no evidence that cryptorchidism is related to being small for gestational age.[25]

The same study showed that 13% of boys born at up to 32 weeks' gestation had undescended testes, compared with 2% of those born after 32 weeks ($p < 0.01$). As birthweight under 1850 g was the criterion for entry to the study, larger infants born after 31 weeks were excluded. In addition, the study suggested a relationship between eczema at 18 months, cryptorchidism and cutaneous steroid use.

4.3 What causes cryptorchidism?

The common causes of cryptorchidism remain essentially unknown. Even though hormones cause testicular descent, hormone deficiency does not appear to be a common cause of undescended testis. This paradox has plagued clinicians and researchers alike for many years. Hormonal deficiences have been sought as an explanation for undescended testis, but most studies have been unable to identify clear-cut hormonal causes. Current knowledge would suggest, therefore, that most undescended testes are caused by mechanical abnormalities. With the recent information about the migration of the gubernaculum and testis from the inguinal region to the scrotum described in Chapter 3, it is quite likely that cryptorchidism most commonly is caused by abnormalities of gubernacular migration. Where true hormonal deficiencies are recognized, i.e. abnormalities of the hypothalamic–pituitary axis or abnormalities of müllerian inhibiting substance secretion, the testes are undescended. However, these defined hormonal syndromes comprise a very small percentage of the total number of children with undescended testes. The common causes of cryptorchidism are listed in Table 4.1.

Table 4.1 Common causes of cryptorchidism

Site of testis	Possible cause
Superficial inguinal pouch	Mechanical failure of gubernacular migration
Ectopic sites	Aberrant gubernacular migration
'Arrested in line of descent'	Hormonal defect in hypothalamic–pituitary–gonadal axis causing failure of gubernacular migration

Failure of the gubernaculum to migrate normally from the inguinal region to the scrotum is likely to account for the common position of an undescended testis in the superficial inguinal pouch. Aberrant migration of the gubernaculum, which is less common, is the likely cause of ectopic testis. Testes which are 'arrested in the line of normal testicular descent' are probably secondary to defects in the hypothalamic–pituitary–gonadal axis or secondary to local abnormalities of testosterone secretion and action.

In most children with undescended testes there is no abnormality of sexual differentiation, suggesting that profound hormonal deficiency is very unlikely as the cause. Although postnatal levels of hormones are diminished in cryptorchidism (as described in Chapter 5), this deficiency postnatally is just as likely to be the effect of malposition at the cause of it.

A wide spectrum of disorders cause cryptorchidism. These include polymalformation syndromes, chromosomal abnormalities, gonadotrophin deficiencies, primary testicular defects, primary neurogenic disorders, and certain mechanical disorders. Many of these categories are interrelated in their causation of undescended testis. A short list of some of the rarer causes of cryptorchidism is shown in the Table 4.2.

Table 4.2 Rare causes of cryptorchidism

Anomaly	Possible cause
Prune belly syndrome	? bladder obstructs inguinal canal
Posterior urethral valves	? bladder obstructs inguinal canal
Persistent müllerian duct syndrome	MIS deficiency/absent MIS receptors
Abdominal wall defects	? decreased abdominal pressure
Spina bifida	genitofemoral nerve dysplasia
Cloacal exstrophy	inguino-scrotal separation
Cerebral palsy	cremaster spasticity
Chromosomal defects	uncertain
Other malformation syndromes	uncertain

MIS = müllerian inhibiting substance.

Numerous inherited or sporadic polymalformation syndromes lead to cryptorchidism. Some of the more common examples include Aarskog's syndrome, Cockayne's syndrome, Frazer syndrome, Lowe syndrome, Smith–Lemli–Opitz syndrome, and sporadic syndromes with undescended testis include Beckwith–Wiedemann syndrome, Cornelia de Lange's syndrome and Noonan's syndrome. Many of these syndromes lead to microcephaly, where pituitary insufficiency or gonadotrophin deficiency also may be related to the cause of undescended testis. Cryptorchidism also occurs with chromosomal derangements, such as trisomy (chromosomes 4, 9, 10, 13, 18, 20, 21) and aneuploidy. These chromosomal anomalies are often associated with prenatal growth deficiency, suggesting hypothalamic adnormalities.

Specific abnormalities of the hypothalamus and pituitary do cause undescended testis. In holoprosencephaly, where the pituitary fails to form, the endocrine glands are small and the testes do not descend. This is caused by profound pituitary hormone deficiency. In pituitary dwarfism with pituitary agenesis and hypogonadism the testes are arrested just below the internal inguinal ring. In the Prader–Willi syndrome, which includes hypogonadotrophism, secondary hypogonadism often is associated with cryptorchidism. Robinow's syndrome often has primary hypogonadism with hypoplastic genitalia and undescended testes.

If the hormone deficiency occurs at puberty rather than in the fetus, as occurs in dystrophia myotonica and Klinefelter's syndrome, the testes are usually fully descended. These syndromes illustrate the importance of the timing of the hormone deficiency with regard to causation of cryptorchidism. In children with complete androgen resistance (testicular feminizing syndrome) the testes are arrested in the inguinal region.

Neurogenic and mechanical abnormalities of fetal development also cause undescended testis. Arthrogryposis multiplex congenita causes joint contractures and absence of muscle, leading to hip dislocation, club foot and scoliosis. The cause of this disorder is unknown, but may be related to abnormalities of the anterior horn cells early in gestation. Bilateral or unilateral undescended testis is common in this syndrome. In a recent review of 57 boys with arthrogryposis multiplex congenita at the Royal Children's Hospital, 18 (32%) had cryptorchidism.[27] Mechanical abnormalities, apart from aberrant gubernacular migration, also can cause undescended testis. External compression of the inguinal region during the last trimester may lead to undescended testis at birth. Our own unpublished data suggest a high incidence of undescended testes in children with dislocated hip and other manifestations of compression *in utero*.

4.4 Cryptorchidism in rare syndromes

There are a number of recognized abnormalities and syndromes in which the incidence of cryptorchidism is significantly higher than in the general population. This section discusses some of those conditions and describes the reasons why they may be associated with cryptorchidism.

4.4.1 Prune belly syndrome

Prune belly syndrome is a rare condition which occurs almost exclusively in boys, and consists of a redundant wrinkled (prune) abdominal wall, dilatation of the entire urinary tract and failure of descent of the testes. Bilateral intra-abdominal testes are a universal finding (Figure 4.9).

For many years prune belly syndrome was thought to be a primary mesodermal defect[28,29] but, in addition to other shortcomings, this concept did not account for the undescended testes. There is now mounting evidence that the cause of prune belly syndrome (PBS) is prenatal urinary obstruction[30–32] although in most cases, no site of obstruction can be identified.[33] We have conjectured that the syndrome is due to a transient obstruction of the urethra between its glandular and penile parts[34] and that this causes gross dilatation of the urinary tract, including the bladder. The degree of distension of the bladder can be documented by ultrasound between 10 and 20 weeks' gestation[35] and

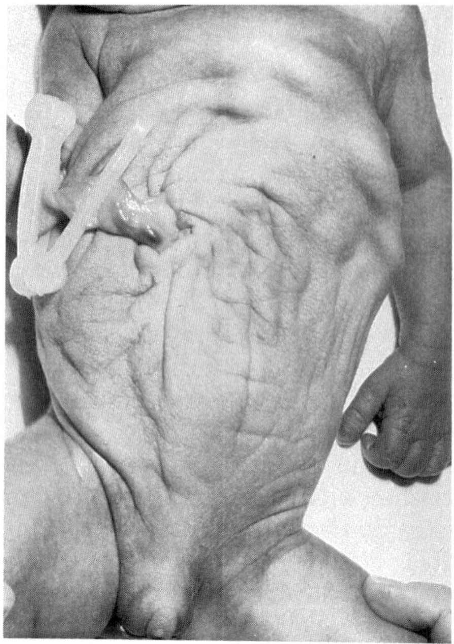

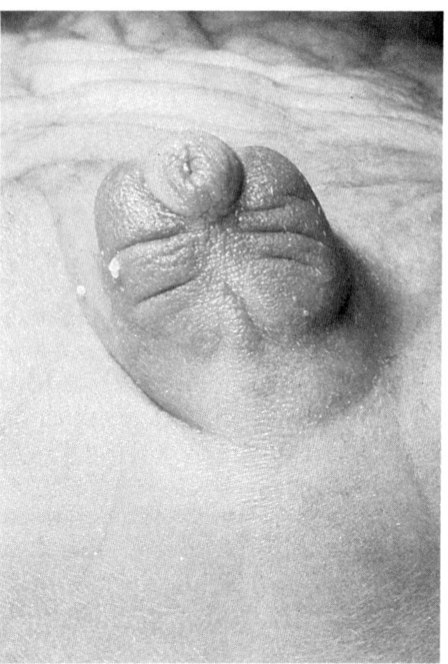

Figure 4.9 Bilateral undescended testes are a universal finding in prune belly syndrome. (a) The wrinkled abdominal wall remains after relief of the gross urinary obstruction *in utero*. (b) The empty, hypoplastic scrotum.

is such that the testes would be prevented from entering the inguinal canal by the peritoneal reflection of the expanding bladder completely obliterating the testes' access to the internal inguinal ring.[34,35] In addition to the separation of the inguinal canal from the peritoneum it is probable, although unproven, that the grossly enlarged bladder causes disruption of the gubernacular apparatus. This would prevent growth of the processus vaginalis into the canal and make it impossible for the testis to descend, even after deflation of the bladder.

The alternative explanation for cryptorchidism in prune belly syndrome[37] is that the syndrome is associated with a low intra-abdominal pressure preventing descent. This is less plausible because the intra-abdominal volume increases during the period of urinary obstruction as a result of the intra-abdominal pressure being markedly increased.[32] After deflation of the bladder with relief of the urinary obstruction, it is probable that the fetus is unable to establish an adequate pressure differential between the abdomen and scrotum, particularly in severe defects where there is gross redundancy of the ventral abdominal wall musculature and ineffective muscular contractions. However, the fact that the processus vaginalis has not been able to develop during the period of bladder distension means that a testis situated at the internal ring would have no patent processus vaginalis down which it can migrate, irrespective of the intra-abdominal pressure.

4.4.2 Posterior urethral valves

Cryptorchidism occurs in 12% of boys with posterior urethral valves.[33] Although this is the only such report linking cryptorchidism and posterior urethral valves, it involved 207 children of whom 24 had undescended testes. Bilateral cryptorchidism occurred in 42%, compared with about 10% in the usual cryptorchid population. The authors suggest that the association may be the result of some common developmental mishap, perhaps of mesenchymal origin. Given the early developmental origin of posterior urethral valves from presumed failure of regression of the urethrovaginal folds of the pelvic urogenital sinus, and the late fetal transinguinal descent of the testis, it is more likely that the high incidence of cryptorchidism occurs because of dilatation of the urinary tract proximal to the urethral obstruction, perhaps in the same way as is seen in the prune belly syndrome.[34]

4.4.3 Exomphalos and gastroschisis

In these conditions there is a defect of the ventral abdominal wall (Figure 4.10) that in males is associated with a high incidence of cryptorchidism.[37,38] The incidence of cryptorchidism at birth and at 1 year in patients with gastroschisis was reported as 18% and 15% respectively, and in those with exomphalos was 52% and 33% respectively.[37] From these data the authors concluded that in male infants there was an association between the abdominal wall defect and cryptorchidism, and that it was consistent with a possible role for intra-abdominal pressure in the process of testicular descent. The inability of the fetus to generate an effective increase in intra-abdominal pressure may have contributed to failure of the testes to enter the inguinal canal and descend normally.[39]

This explanation has not been accepted universally: for example, Hadziselimovic believes that the presence of concomitant brain malformations[38] is significant, and causes the cryptorchidism. Some of these malformations of the brain described, e.g. spina bifida, themselves have a potentially independent effect on testicular descent (see Section 4.4.4) There is no direct evidence that the association described relates to disruption of the hypothalamic–pituitary–gonadal axis, as suggested by Hadziselimovic *et al.*[38]

4.4.4 Spina bifida

Until 1981, cryptorchidism was not recognized as a significant problem in children with meningomyelocele,[40] although many clinicians may

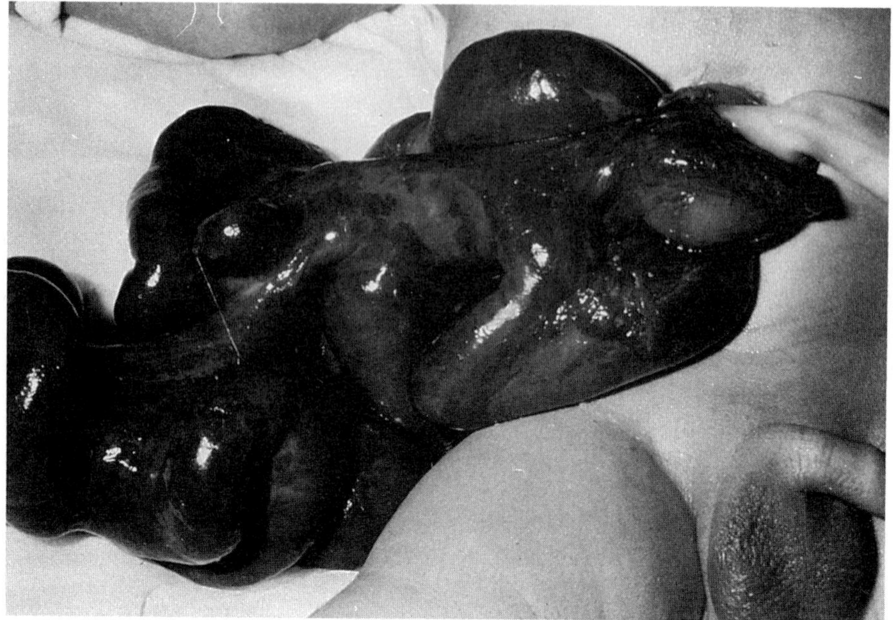

Figure 4.10 Gastroschisis is commonly associated with undescended testes, which occasionally may herniate through the defect. In this infant, both testes are descended.

have suspected the incidence of undescended testes in boys with spina bifida to be higher than that of the normal population. Kropp and Voeller observed cryptorchidism in 6 of 23 boys with spina bifida.

In two other recent studies,[41,42] a similarly high incidence of cryptorchidism has been reported in spina bifida: combined with our own patients, this represents 15 out of 85 boys (18%) with undescended testes.

The level of the sensory and motor deficit affected the incidence of undescended testes, and lesions above L2 were found to have a greater association with cryptorchidism. Disruption of nerve root and spinal cord function in spina bifida is not always clear cut or predictable in relation to the external appearance of the lesion or to its level, which may account for the variability of the observations.[43] Nevertheless, it would seem that the incidence of undescended testes is increased significantly in spina bifida, particularly where the lesion is at or above L3.

The most compelling evidence comes from the computerized data from the International Myelodysplasia Project, Seattle through the kind assistance of David Shurtleff, MD. Of the 470 boys included in the file, the position of the testes and the level of the spina bifida lesion were recorded in 345, and 81 (23%) had undescended testes. Undescended testes were present, both unilateral and bilateral, in 19% (37 out of 186) of the low lesions, compared with 21 out of 59 (36%) in the high lumbar area (see Figure 3.9, page 42) These data strongly support the proposal that abnormalities of the high lumbar cord are associated with a significant increase in cryptorchidism.

4.4.5 Cloacal exstrophy (Figure 4.11)

Postmortem examination of an infant born with cloacal exstrophy has provided some clues to a possible mechanism of failure of testicular descent in this condition.[44] On each side an intra-abdominal testis was

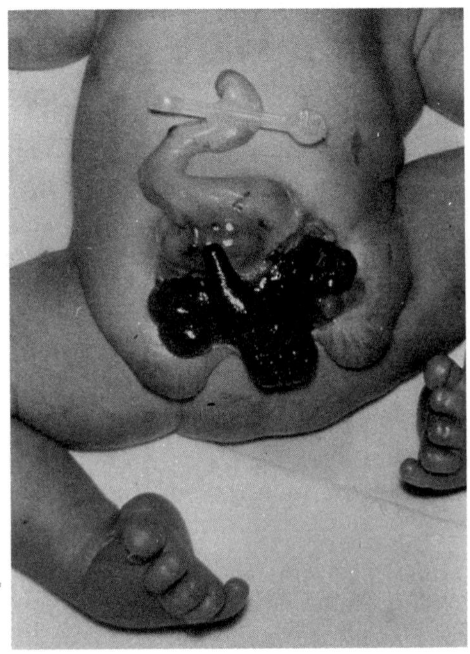

Figure 4.11 Cloacal exstrophy associated with bilateral intra-abdominal testes.

attached by the gubernaculum to an evertable pouch in the lateral abdominal wall. The internal ring was located at the site of the pouch. Despite the severe pubic diastasis, the scrotum was located medially, far removed from the laterally placed inguinal canal. Each testis could be manipulated into the base of its pouch but was prevented from descending further by the tough fascia of the flank which separated it from the scrotum (Figure 4.12).

The testes apparently failed to descend beyond the inguinal canal because of their abnormal position. The tight fascial planes replacing the low-pressure scrotal space outside the external ring may have prevented

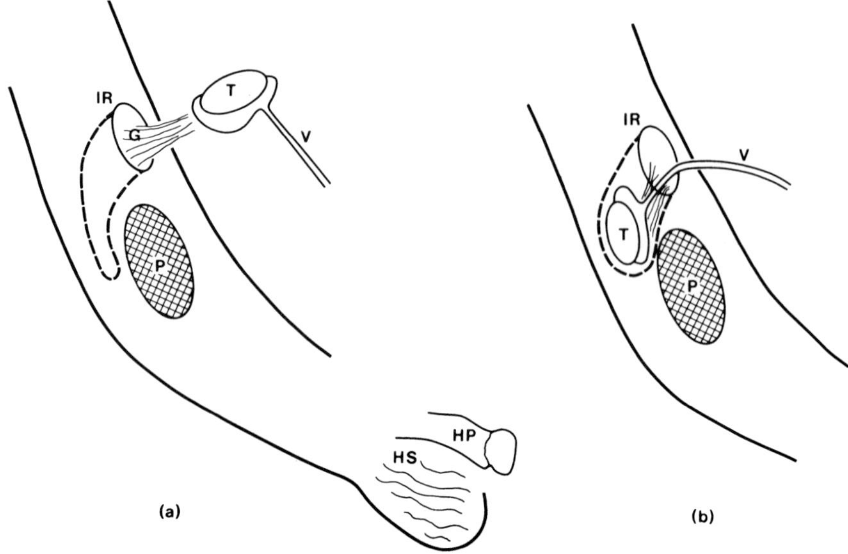

Figure 4.12 The anatomy found in a boy with cloacal exstrophy. (a) Testis (T) in an intra-abdominal position attached to the internal ring (IR) by a peritoneal fold containing gubernaculum (G). (b) The testis could be evaginated into the pouch to recreate the normal anatomy of the inguinal canal (V = vas; P = pubis; HP = hemipenis; HS = hemiscrotum). (Reproduced with permission from Reference 4.)

descent. This clinical example of mechanical failure of descent supports the hypothesis that a pressure gradient across the inguinal canal is required for normal descent to occur.[10,45] This is consistent with the observation that external compression can delay testicular descent in rodents.[46]

4.4.6 Cerebral palsy

Several studies have shown that the incidence of 'cryptorchidism' in cerebral palsy is higher than expected.[47–49] The overall prevalence of cryptorchidism in postpubertal males with cerebral palsy is reported as ranging from 41%[48] to 53.8%.[49] Although several possible aetiologies for these findings have been offered previously, including anomalies of the gubernaculum, Leydig cell atrophy and decreased luteinizing hormone response to luteinizing hormone-releasing factor, none of these has been demonstrated consistently in cerebral palsy.

The fact that there is no evidence that damage to the fetal hypothalamic-pituitary-gonadal axis occurs at a stage that would interfere with normal testicular descent has resulted in a search for alternative mechanisms to account for the observed phenomena.[50] One feature of cerebral palsy is the progressive spasticity of muscles with increasing age.[51,52] There is often little evidence of spasticity in infants at the time of diagnosis. Many muscle groups have been incriminated, and it would seem likely that the cremaster muscle also could be involved. This involvement would lead to increased cremasteric spasm and a relatively higher position of the testis with growth.

To test this possibility, boys with an unequivocal diagnosis of cerebral palsy were compared with age-matched controls selected from within the general inpatient population.[53] In infants with cerebral palsy, the testes were on average 5.2 ± 1.2 cm (mean ± SD) below the pubic tubercle compared with 6.1 ± 0.8 cm in the children in the age-matched control group (Figure 4.13) In 5–10-year-old children with cerebral palsy, the testes

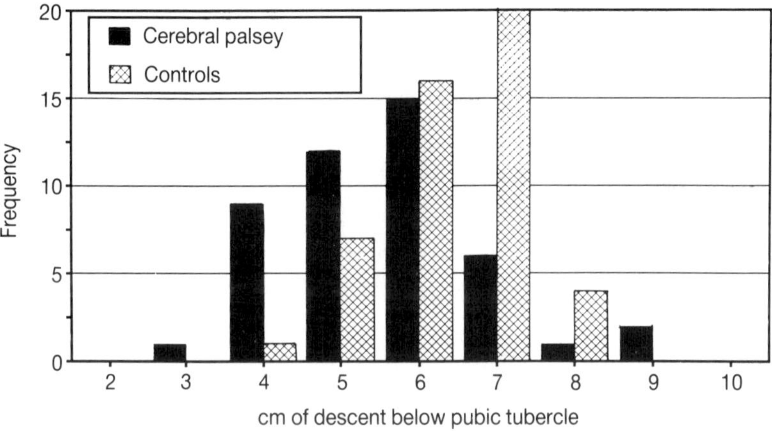

Figure 4.13 Cryptorchidism in infants less than 30 months of age. The position of the testis in centimetres below the pubic tubercle is recorded against the frequency, for infants with cerebral palsy versus normal infants. (Reproduced with permission from Reference 51.)

remained in a similar position, 5.6 ± 1.4 cm, whereas in the children in the age-matched control group the testes were significantly lower (7.3 ± 1.3 cm) (Figure 4.14). While the testes remained the same distance below the pubis in cerebral palsy, the distance increased significantly in normal children.

These data suggest that there may be no prenatal interference with descent in cerebral palsy; but rather, the cremaster muscle, which may become spastic during childhood, causes secondary ascent of the testis and/or prevents elongation of the spermatic cord with growth. This hypothesis suggests that the incidence of 'cryptorchidism' would appear to increase during childhood as spasticity increases. These data would fit with the observations of Rundle *et al.*[47] and Cortada and Kousseff,[48] that in

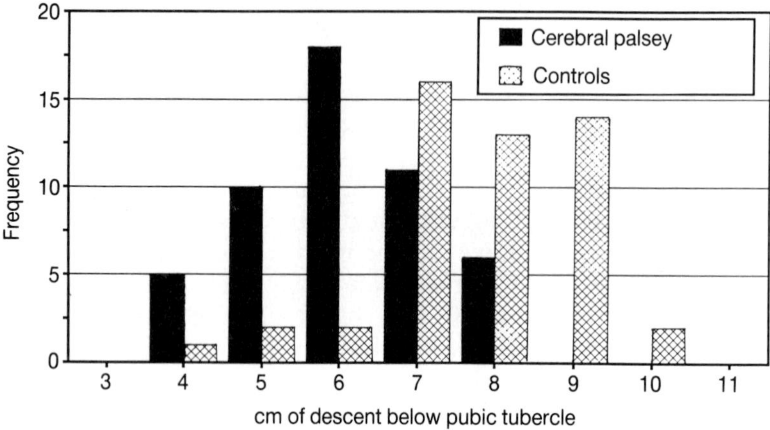

Figure 4.14 Cryptorchidism in children between 5 and 10 years of age. The position of the testis in centimetres below the pubic tubercle is plotted against the frequency, for normal boys versus boys with cerebral palsy. (Reproduced with permission from Reference 53.)

older children and adults, the apparent incidence of cryptorchidism may reach 50%.

4.4.7 Testicular–epididymal fusion abnormalities

A number of testicular–epididymal fusion abnormalities have been described (Figure 4.15).[54] These abnormalities may contribute to the higher rate of infertility seen in adults who had undescended testes during childhood.

All descriptions of epididymal abnormalities report a high incidence of concomitant cryptorchidism.[55–57] The comparative incidence in boys with normally descended testes is not known for certain, but is believed to be low. Abnormalities range from simple epididymal elongation to complete separation of the epididymis and testis.[55] The higher the arrest of testicular descent, the more abnormal the associated ductal system tends to be.[58]

Where there is a severe epididymal abnormality or complete separation of the two structures, as is most commonly observed in intra-abdominal or intracanicular testis, the (as yet unresolved) question which must be asked is whether it would be appropriate to remove the gonad in this situation, as sperm transport is bound to be affected.[59] Early successful orchidopexy alone may not ensure subsequent fertility despite the presence of normal germ cells.[58]

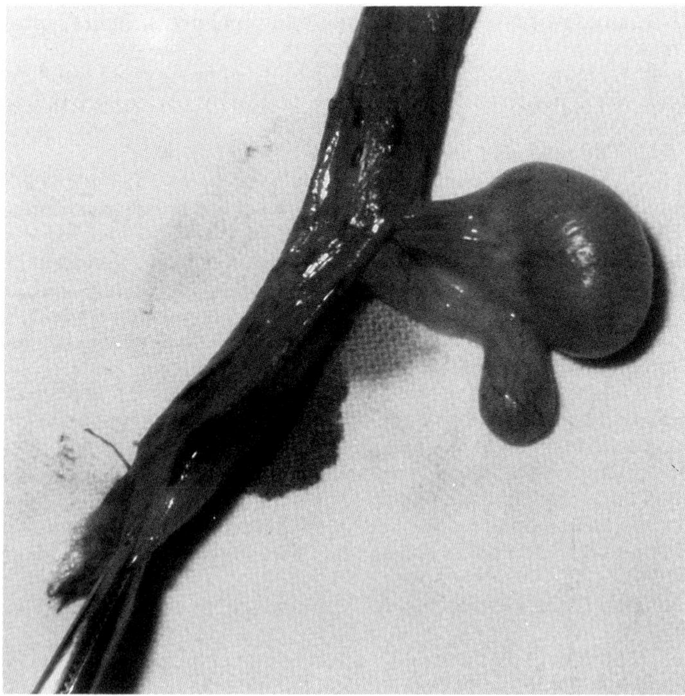

Figure 4.15 Partial separation of the testis and epididymis as seen at orchidopexy. Here the caudal epididymis is detached from the lower pole of the testis, although the rete testis is intact.

References

1. Wyllie GG. The diagnosis of undescended testes. *Med J Aust* 1978; **1:** 639–41.
2. Jones PG. Undescended testes. *Aust. Paediatr. J* 1966; **2:** 36–48.
3. Browne D. The diagnosis of undescended testicle. *Br Med J* 1938; **ii:** 168.
4. Scorer CG, Farrington GH. *Congenital Deformities of the Testis and Epididymis.* London: Butterworths, 1971.
5. Thevasthasan CG. Transverse ectopia of the testis. *Aust NZ J Surg* 1967; **37:** 93–102.
6. Beasley SW, Auldist AW. Crossed testicular ectopia in association with double incomplete testicular descent. *Aust NZ J Surg* 1985; **55:** 301–3.
7. Gauderer MW, Grisoni ER, Stellato TA, Ponsky JL, Izant RJ Jr. Transverse testicular ectopia. *J Pediatr Surg* 1982; **17:** 43–7.
8. Doraiswamy NV. Crossed ectopic testis – case report and review. *Z Kinderchir* 1983; **38:** 264–8.
9. Hutson JM, Chow CW, Ng WD. Persistent müllerian duct syndrome with transverse testicular ectopia. *Pediatr Surg Int* 1987; **2:** 191–4.
10. Frey HL, Rajfer J. Role of the gubernaculum and intra-abdominal pressure in the process of testicular descent. *J Urol* 1984; **131:** 574–9.

11. Attah AA, Hutson JM. The role of intraabdominal pressure in cryptorchidism. 1992 (In press).
12. Farrington GH. The position and retractability of the normal testis in childhood with reference to the diagnosis and treatment of cryptorchidism. *J Pediatr Surg* 1968; **3:** 53–9.
13. Wyllie GG. The retractile testis. *Med J Aust* 1984; **140:** 403–5.
14. Atwell JD. Ascent of the testis. Fact or fiction. *Br J Urol* 1985; **57:** 474–7.
15. Fenton ED, Woodward AA, Hudson IL, Marschner I. The ascending testis. *Pediatr Surg Int* 1990; **4:** 6–9.
16. (a) John Radcliffe Hospital Cryptorchidism Study Group. Cryptorchidism: an apparent substantial increase since 1960. *Br Med J* 1986; **293:** 1401–4.
(b) John Radcliffe Hospital Cryrptorchidism Study Group. Boys with late descending testes: the source of patients with 'retractile' testes undergoing orchidopexy. *Br Med J* 1986; **293:** 789–90.
17. Scorer CG. The descent of the testis. *Arch Dis Child* 1964; **39:** 605–9.
18. Bishop PMF. Studies in clinical endocrinology. V. The management of the undescended testis. *Guys Hosp Rep* 1945; **94:** 12–74.
19. Nelson WO. Some problems of testicular function. *J Urol* 1953; **69:** 325–8.
20. Campbell HE. Incidence of malignant growth of the undescended testicle: a critical and statistical study. *Arch Surg* 1942; **44:** 353–69.
21. Baumrucker GO. Incidence of testicular pathology. *Bull US Army Med Dept* 1946; **5:** 312.
22. Coldony AH. Undescended testes – is surgery necessary? *N Engl J Med* 1986; **314:** 510–11.
23. Pike MC, Chilvers C, Peckham MJ. Effect of age at orchidopery on risk of testicular cancer. *The Lancet* 1986; I: 1246–8.
24. MacKellar A, Lugg MM, Keogh EJ (1984) The undescended testis: lies, damned lies and statistics. In: Kalami, Pryor, eds. *Progress in Reproductive Biology and Medicine*. Basel: Karger, 1984: Vol. 10, pp. 24–30.
25. Morley R, Lucas A. Undescended testes in low birthweight infants. *Br Med J* 1987; **295:** 753.
26. Fonkalsrud EW, Mengel W (1981) *The Undescended Testis*. Chicago: Year Book Medical Publishers, 1981.
27. Fallat ME, Williams MPL, Farmer P, Hutson JM. Histologic evaluation of inguinoscrotal migration of the gubernaculum in rodents during testicular descent and its relationship to the genitofemoral nerve. *Pediatr Surg Int* (1992) (In press).
28. Nunn P, Stephens FD. The triad syndrome: a composite anomaly of the abdominal wall, urinary system and testes. *J Urol* 1961; **86:** 782–94.
29. Wigger HJ, Blanc WA. The prune belly syndrome. *Pathol Annu* 1977; **1:** 17–39.
30. Adzick NS, Harrison MR, Flake AW, De Lorimer AA. Urinary extravasation in the fetus with obstructive uropathy. *J Pediatr Surg* 1985; **20:** 608–15.
31. Moerman P, Fryns JP, Goddeeris P, Lauweryns JM. Pathogenesis of the prune belly syndrome: A fractional urethral obstruction caused by prostatic hypoplasia. *Pediatrics* 1984; **73:** 470–5.
32. Pagon RA, Smith DW, Shephard TH. Urethral obstruction malformation complex: a cause of abdominal muscle deficiency and the 'prune belly'. *J Pediatr* 1979; **94:** 900–6.
33. Kreuger RP, Hardy BE, Churchill BM. Cryptorchidism in boys with posterior urethral valves. *J Urol* 1980; **124:** 101–2.
34. Hutson JM, Beasley SW. The aetiology of prune belly syndrome. *Aust Paediatr J* 1987; **23:** 309.
35. Anderson JC, Faulder KG, Mpor JE. 'Prune belly' syndrome. *Med J Aust* 1979; **i:** 314–5.

36. Beasley SW, Bettenay F, Hutson JM. The anterior urethra provides clues to the aetiology of prune belly syndrome. *Pediatr Surg Int* 1988; **3:** 169–72.
37. Kaplan LM, Koyle MA, Kaplan GW, Farrer JH, Rajfer J. Association between abdominal wall defect and cryptorchidism. *J Urol* 1986; **136:** 645.
38. Hadziselimovic F, Duckett JW, Snyder II HM, Schnaufer L, Huff D. Omphalocele, cryptorchidism and brain malformations. *J Pediatr Surg* 1987; **22:** 854–6.
39. Quinlan DM, Gearhart JP, Jeffs RD. Abdominal wall defects and cryptorchidism: an animal model. *J Urol* 1988; **140:** 1141–4.
40. Kropp KA, Voeller KKA. Cryptorchidism in meningomyelocele. *J Pediatr* 1981; **99:** 110–3.
41. Meyer S, Landau H. Precocious puberty in myelomeningocele patients. *J Paedtr Orthoped.* 1984; **4:** 28–3.
42. Greene SA, Frank M, Zachmann M *et al.* Growth and sexual development in children with myelomeningocele. *Eur J Pediatr* 1985; **144:** 146–8.
43. Barson AJ. Developmental pathology of the spine. In: Davis JA, Dobbing J, *Scientific Foundations of Pediatrics.* (ed 2). London: Heinemann, 1981: 2nd edn, pp. 759–85.
44. Hutson JM, Beasley SW. Why testicular descent may be impaired in cloacal exstrophy. *Pediatr Surg Int* 1989; **4:** 122–3.
45. Frey HL, Peng S, Raijfer J. Synergy of abdominal pressure and androgens in testicular descent. *Biol Reprod* 1983; **29:** 1233–9.
46. Luthra M, Hutson JM, Stephens FD. Effects of external inguinoscrotal compression on descent of the testis in rats. *Pediatr Surg Int* 1989; **4:** 403–7.
47. Rundle JSH, Primrose DA, Carachi R. Cryptorchidism in cerebral palsy. *Br J Urol* 1982; **54:** 170–1.
48. Cortada X, Kousseff BG. Cryptorchidism in mental retardation. *J Urol* 1984; **131:** 674–6.
49. Ankerhold J, Gressmann C. Hodendescensustorungen beim frukindlichen Hirschaden. *Z Kinderchir* 1969; **107:** 15–25.
50. Hutson JM, Beasley SW. Embryological controversies in testicular descent. *Semin Urol* 1988; **6:** 68–73.
51. St-Anne Dargassies S. Neurodevelopmental symptoms during the first year of life. *Dev Med Child Neurol* 1984; **14:** 235–6.
52. McLellan L. Therapeutic possibilities in cerebral palsy: A neurologist's view. *Clin Dev Med* 1984; **90:** 97–8.
53. Smith JA, Hutson JM, Beasley SW, Reddihough DS. The relationship between cerebral palsy and cryptorchidism. *J Pediatr Surg* 1989; **23:** 275–7.
54. Toth J, Merksz M, Szonyi P. States causing infertility in adulthood in children with undescended testes. *Acta Chirurg Hungarica* 1987; **28:** 243–6.
55. Koff WJ, Scaletscky R. Malformations of the epididymis in undescended testis. *J Urol* 1990; **143:** 340–3.
56. Heath AL, Man DW, Eckstein HB. Epididymal abnormalities associated with maldescent of the testis. *J Pediatr Surg* 1984; **19:** 47–9.
57. Johansen TEB. Anatomy of the testis and epididymis in cryptorchidism. *Andrologia* 1987; **19:** 565–9.
58. Gill B, Kogan S, Starr S, Reda E, Levitt S. Significance of epididymal and ductal anomalies associated with testicular maldescent. *J Urol* 1989; **142:** 556–8.
59. Belman AB. Editorial comment. *J Urol* 1990; **143:** 343.

5

The postnatal effects of cryptorchidism

5.1 A primary anomaly or secondary effects?

Since John Hunter first took a scientific interest in undescended testes and the mechanism of testicular descent, it has been uncertain whether the testis is primarily abnormal leading to maldescent, or alternatively is undescended and becomes secondarily abnormal (Figure 5.1). Because 'undescended testis' comprises a heterogeneous group of conditions, including some that have known primary abnormalities of the testes, it is not always easy to separate primary causes from secondary effects.

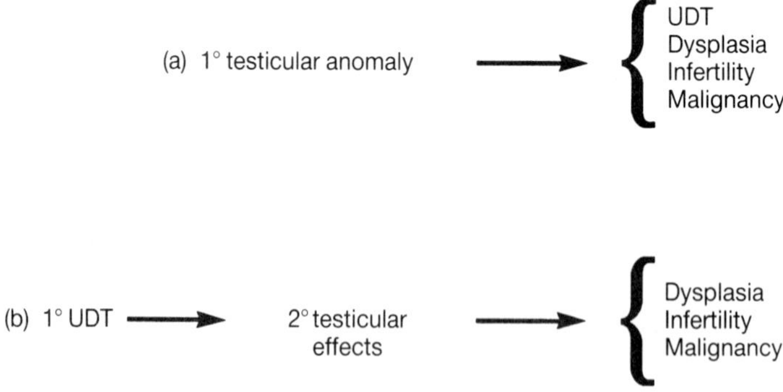

Figure 5.1 Schemas showing the two main theories to explain the testicular dysplasia in undescended testes. (a) One theory is that maldescent and testicular dysplasia are both caused by a primary defect in testicular development. (b) The alternative theory is that a normal testis fails to descend, and the high temperature leads to secondary dysplasia.

A growing body of evidence suggests that many of the abnormalities seen postnatally in cryptorchidism are secondary, although occasional primary abnormalities in the hypothalamic–pituitary–gonadal axis may lead to inadequate hormone secretion from the testes and subsequent maldescent. Giwercman *et al.*[1] postulated that tumours arise in undescended testes because of a primary anomaly. In this chapter we will discuss the documented abnormalities seen postnatally in cryptorchidism on the premise that they are more likely to be secondary abnormalities, although some may still be proven to be primary in origin.

Differences in the results of animal and human studies have been a complicating factor in unravelling the effects of undescended testis. Many studies on the effects of cryptorchidism have been performed on the laboratory rat, in which the important developmental aspects of gubernacular migration are complete by 10 days after birth, but the testis does not descend into the scrotum until the onset of puberty, at 3–4 weeks. This is in sharp contrast to the human where gubernacular and testicular descent occur simultaneously before birth (see figure 3.2, page 34). Most effects of undescended testes in the rat, therefore, do not become evident until after puberty: at best, this makes extrapolation of results in the rat awkward, and at worst, impossible.

Another problem in analysing the effects of undescended testes is the separation of the effects in true cryptorchid testes from those in retractile testes. As will be detailed below, the possible effects of retractile testes are controversial, with some studies demonstrating retractile testes to be significantly abnormal while others suggest that they are normal.

5.1.1 The effect of temperature

The secondary effects seen in undescended testes are believed to be caused by the increased temperature of the undescended testis compared with its scrotal counterpart. The scrotal testis resides in a specialized low-temperature environment with heat exchange mechanisms in the pampiniform plexus, pigmentation of the scrotal skin, absence of subcutaneous fat, and regulation by temperature-sensitive muscles, i.e. the cremaster and dartos muscles (Figure 5.2).[2] In the human, the scrotal testis is at 33°C compared with an inguinal testis which is at approximately 35°C and the intra abdominal testis at 37°C.[2] On an evolutionary time scale, the testis has descended into this specialized external, low-temperature environment for advantages in sperm storage, particularly in the epididymis.[3] The one hundred and twenty million years that has elapsed since the testis first descended in primitive mammals has allowed ample time for adaptation of the physiological mechanism within the testis to this special environment. It is not surprising, therefore, that in undescended testes the secondary increase in their ambient temperature leads to their progressive dysfunction. Most enzymes and cellular mechanisms within the testes

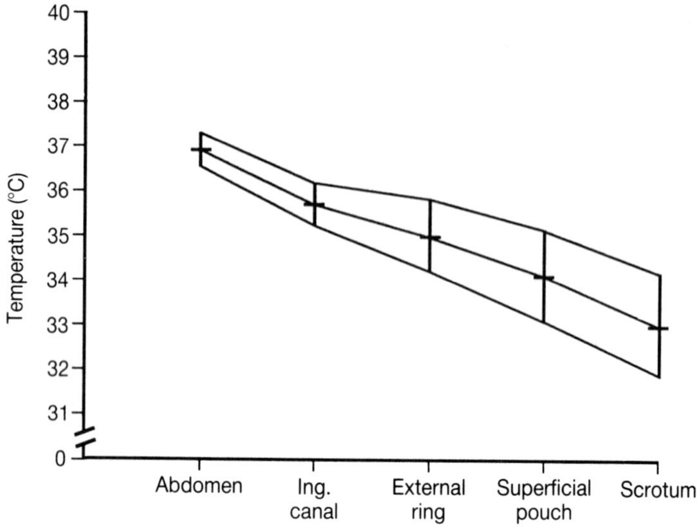

Figure 5.2 The temperatures (mean ± SD) of the various sites where the testis may be found, showing that the scrotum is a specialized low-temperature environment. (Adapted and redrawn from Reference 2.)

appear to be well-adapted to this lower-than-normal body temperature.[4] Indeed, this reference from Steinberger comes from a recent international meeting on the detrimental effects of temperature on the testis.[5]

5.2 Endocrine effects

Studies in the rat

Studies of rats made cryptorchid by operation before the onset of puberty show no gross abnormalities in the steroidogenic pathways in the testes, and indicate that the mechanism of action of hCG on the Leydig cells is unaffected by this procedure.[6] Attempts to replicate the human situation with undescended testes from birth have been conducted by making rats surgically cryptorchid in the first few days after birth. The intratesticular content of testosterone in the descended testis rises from low levels of 0.3 ng per testis at two weeks of age to over 70 ng per testis at 1½ months. By contrast, in the undescended testis the intratesticular testosterone content is normal at 2 weeks but fails to rise after puberty, reaching only 2ng per testis at 1½ months.[7] The same authors have measured the activity of testosterone biosynthetic enzymes in the cryptorchid testes and have found that these enzymes are inhibited at 1½ months of age to levels less than 20% of the normal value. They concluded that in undescended testes there was deficient testosterone synthesis from the Leydig cells after puberty and that this may account for subsequent morphological abnormalities and infertility.

The physiology of the adult rat testis which has been made cryptorchid at birth is deranged such that gonadotrophic regulation of both Leydig and Sertoli cells is abnormal.[8] Bergh and co-authors[9] in a study of the rat made unilaterally cryptorchid at birth, found significant reduction in the weight of the adult testes but normal numbers of Sertoli and Leydig cells. The number of LH, FSH and prolactin receptors were all reduced in the intra-abdominal testis. By contrast, the number of LHRH receptors was unaffected. In addition, testosterone concentrations were decreased in the intra-abdominal testis. In a related study[10] abnormalities in Sertoli and Leydig cell function at 20 days of age, the time when the contralateral testes would be descending, were demonstrated. These very early endocrine abnormalities appear to precede subsequent morphological abnormalities.

Many authors have studied the hormonal effects of cryptorchidism produced by surgery in adult rats.[11] LH levels in the cryptorchid adult are increased within 1 week of operation and remain so; a similar increase in serum FSH levels occurs.[12] The testicular content of testosterone decreased in the cryptorchid testis while it increased in the normal contralateral testis. The levels of oestrogen receptors within the testis increased. These results demonstrate that the cryptorchid adult testis has diminished steroidogenic capacity, but that the Leydig cells remain viable.[13] Bilateral cryptorchidism in rats or sheep interferes in subtle ways with the negative feedback on the pituitary, such that the microheterogeneity in the isoelectric variants of LH is disturbed.[14]

Functional derangements in Sertoli cells after cryptorchidism have been documented in a number of reports, and these are summarized by de Kretzer and Risbridger.[15] Production of seminiferous tubule fluid, secretion of androgen-binding protein and inhibin production, are all suppressed after experimental cryptorchidism in adults. The increase in tubule fluid seen in sexually mature rats made cryptorchid at birth, is at odds with the effects in mature rats. The exact derangement produced by cryptorchidism depends, therefore, on the degree of testicular development in ways that as yet remain unknown.

5.2.2. Hormonal levels in human studies.

Early attempts to measure LH and FSH in humans with undescended testes[16] showed that LH serum levels were normal in cryptorchid boys whereas some had evaluated FSH levels. They speculated that elevated FSH may correlate with deranged testicular function, while elevated LH occurred only when the gonad was absent. Koch and Rahlf[17] performed LHRH stimulation tests on boys with undescended testes and compared them with a control group that had undergone previous surgery for cryptorchidism. They found about 80% of the prepubertal boys had low or normal basal levels of LH while 20% had elevated levels. They concluded that this variable response to gonadotrophin indicated a heterogeneous group of patients.

In 1976 Walsh *et al.*[18] performed hCG-stimulation tests on boys with undescended testes. They found that the gonadotrophin-dependent phase of testosterone production was present and that the hCG-stimulation test was unable to detect abnormalities in boys with unilateral cryptorchidism. In a cross-sectional study of 168 boys with cryptorchidism urinary testosterone excretion was elevated in boys who were under 9 years of age.[19] The normal pubertal increase in testosterone excretion was moderately delayed in these patients although later in puberty the testosterone secretion was normal. It was concluded that disturbances in the hypothalamic–pituitary gonadal axis in children with undescended testes might be present during early childhood.

Gendrel *et al.*[20] have examined the plasma gonadotrophin and testosterone levels in infants with undescended testes (Figure 5.3). In approximately half these infants, the testes descended spontaneously between 2 and 4 months. (Now we would call these 'ascending' testes, as described in Chapter 4.) In those children in which the testes remained undescended, the postnatal rise in the plasma LH level and testosterone concentrations were significantly lower than normal, and there was a correlation between the plasma LH and testosterone levels. They postulated an abnormality in LH secretion as the cause for cryptorchidism

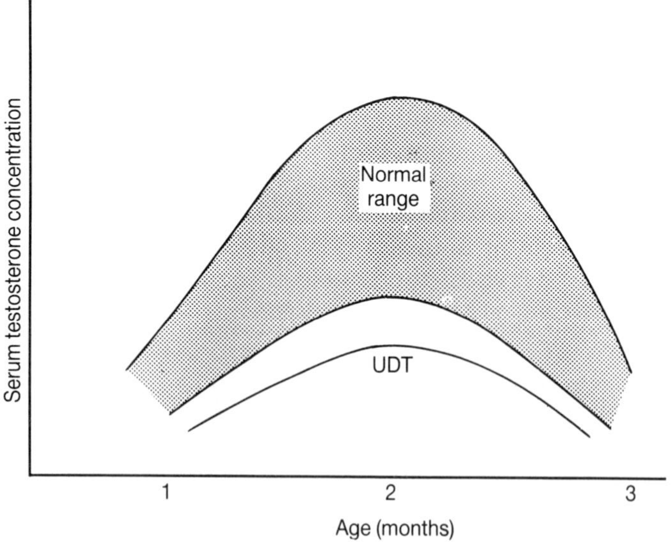

Figure 5.3 Schema showing the postnatal peak in serum testosterone levels between 1 and 3 months in normal boys and those with undescended testes. (Adapted and redrawn from Reference 20.)

leading to a deficient postnatal surge of testosterone. Whether their documented androgen deficiency postnatally is a primary abnormality or a secondary effect of the undescended testes is not yet resolved. A detailed account of steroidogenesis in normal and cryptorchid boys is provided by Jockenhovel and Swerdloff,[21] to which the reader is referred.

Van Vliet *et al.*[22] investigated 40 prepubertal boys with LHRH-stimulation tests. They found an increase in basal FSH levels and an increase in FSH response to LHRH in both unilateral and bilaterally cryptorchid boys. The FSH receptor levels-per-testis were lower in the undescended testis than in the normally descended testis.[23] The level of LH receptors was also found to be significantly inhibited.

Baker *et al.*[24] looked at premature infants born with a mean gestational age of thirty weeks. Although some testes descended postnatally, there was a persisting high incidence (up to 19%) of undescended testes at eighteen months of age. The normal testosterone surge in the second postnatal month failed to develop in the premature babies with subsequently proven cryptorchidism. In addition, these premature babies failed to show an immediate postnatal testosterone peak which is normally seen in association with residual hCG in the neonatal circulation. They concluded that inadequate stimulation of testosterone by hCG *in utero* may contribute to the pathogenesis of undescended testis in this special group of premature babies.

In a detailed study of androgen levels in infancy, Job *et al.*[25] found significantly decreased plasma testosterone levels and LH levels from 1 to 4 months of age. After 4 months of age, the normal LH and testosterone levels were very low, and no differences could be documented between cryptorchid infants and normal children. They found antibodies against gonadotrophin-producing cells in the pituitary on immunofluorescence in half the infants with undescended testes, and speculated that maternal auto-antibodies may be responsible for partial gonadotrophin deficiency in the perinatal period, leading to undescended testes in the male offspring. In these very small infants FSH basal levels and levels in response to LHRH were found to be within the normal range.

5.2.3 Androgen receptor levels

Androgen receptor levels in scrotal skin fibroblasts and cells from testicular biopsies taken at orchidopexy are normal in boys with bilateral undescended testes.[26]

5.2.4 Müllerian inhibiting substance (MIS)

Recent studies from our own laboratory utilizing an enzyme immunoassay for MIS show a peak of secretion between four and twelve months of age (Figure 5.4).[27] MIS peak levels are therefore occurring after the postnatal

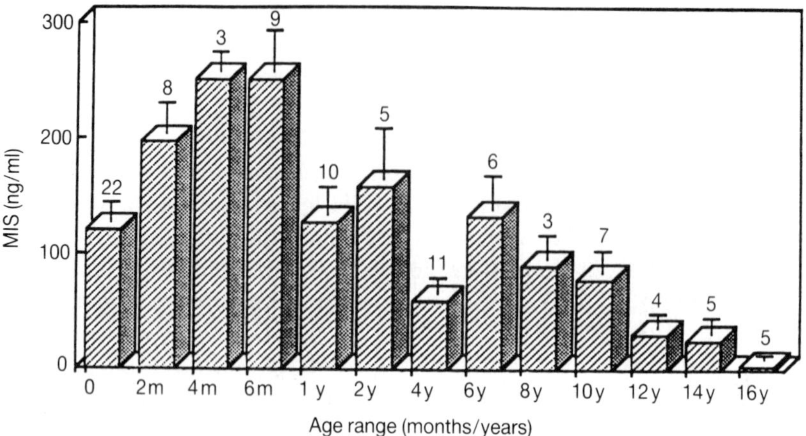

Figure 5.4 Mean (± SE) serum müllerian inhibiting substance (MIS) levels at different ages. Note the peak of secretion from 4 to 12 months. (Reproduced with permission from Reference 27.)

surge of androgen secretion between 1 and 4 months of age.[25] When levels of MIS in normal children were compared with those undergoing orchidopexy, a deficient surge of MIS secretion between 4 and 12 months of age was documented (Figure 5.5).[28] In later years of childhood, there was a measurable but not always statistically significant inhibition in MIS levels in boys with undescended testes. Importantly, in the first 3 months of life no deficiency of MIS secretion could be documented in the small number of cases measured. This would be consistent with the later depression in MIS secretion being a secondary rather than a primary abnormality.

5.3 Morphological effects

5.3.1. Animal studies

Experimental cryptorchidism leads to a wide range of morphological changes in the testes. After neonatal transection of the gubernaculum in rats, the first change is an increase in the lipid content of the Sertoli cells at day 16. Subsequently there is dilatation of the cisternae of the smooth endoplastic reticulum and changes in the cell–cell junctional complexes.[15] The volumetric density of Leydig cells increased over three-fold after cryptorchidism was produced, consistent with important changes in Sertoli–Leydig cell interactions.[15] These authors postulate the morphological changes are consequent upon local alterations in the paracrine mechanisms within the testis.

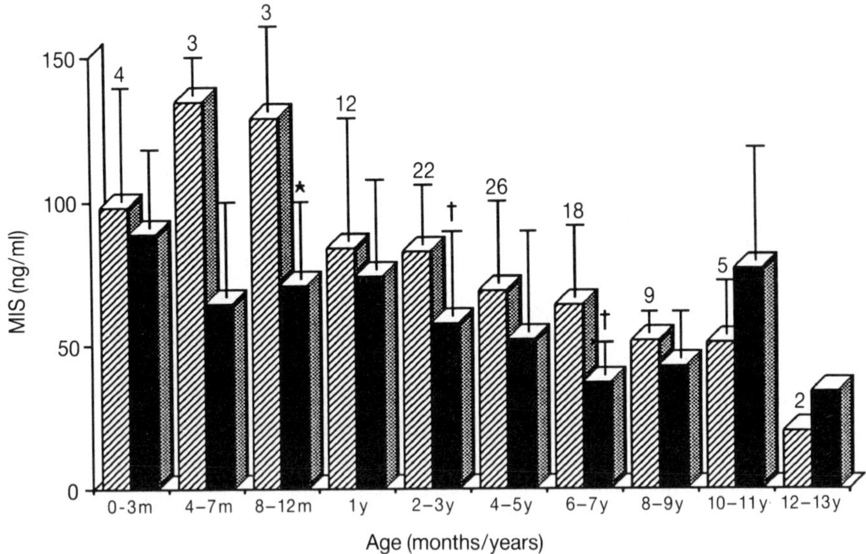

Figure 5.5 Mean (±SD) serum müllerian inhibiting substance (MIS) levels in boys with undescended testes (■) and paired, age-matched controls (▨). Note the lack of a peak of secretion at 4 to 12 months in boys with undescended testes. (Reproduced with permission from Reference 28.)

5.3.2 Human studies

It was once thought that morphological abnormalities within the undescended testis, i.e. germinal cell deficiency, were congenital.[29] In recent years, however, it has been observed that the testicular morphology is normal initially and becomes abnormal as childhood progresses. The first macroscopic changes are seen in 5–10 year-olds, where the testis may be small and softer than normal. Histologically, they show signs of dysplasia. In 1974, Mengel *et al.*[30] reported on a large histological study of 752 testicular biopsy specimens from children between 2 months and 15 years of age. They counted the number of spermatogonia observed in 50 tubules and measured the diameter of the tubules and were unable to identify abnormalities in the first or second year of life. By contrast, in the third year of life they found a significant fall in the number of the spermatogonia per tubule, and a lack of the normal enlargement of the tubules. Similar but less severe abnormalities were observed in the unilaterally descended testes at a later age. They concluded that to prevent this apparently secondary effect on testicular morphology, orchidopexy should be performed before the second birthday.

Hadziselimovic *et al.*[31] performed electron-microscopic studies on testicular biopsies collected at orchidopexy. They found no ultrastructural abnormalities in the tubules before the first birthday, although there were early abnormalities in the Leydig cells. They concluded that the optimal time for surgical intervention was in the second year of life. Hadziselimovic *et al.* published detailed accounts of their histological studies in the mid-1980s.[32] They found that development of the Leydig cells between 2 and 6 months was impaired in undescended testes, whereas the Sertoli cells and germ cells appeared normal. Around 6 months of age the normal transformation of gonocytes into spermatogonia (Figure 5.6) was completed, and the number of germ cells begins to diminish significantly, even in normal boys.

By the end of the second year of life, they found that nearly 40% of all undescended testes have completely lost their germ cells. The severity of germ cell deficiency is directly related to the position of the testis, with higher or intra-abdominal testes being more severely abnormal than testes located just outside the scrotum. Hadziselimovic concluded that germ cell deficiency in undescended testes is a secondary abnormality. In undescended testes examined by biopsy, only one infant in 92 younger than 12 months of age lacked all germ cells, and that 70% of the testicular biopsies examined had a normal number of germ cells.[33] In animal experiments germ cell deficiency and arrest of spermatogenesis may be reversible, since studies on lambs show recovery of germ cell numbers and spermatogenesis after orchidopexy.[34]

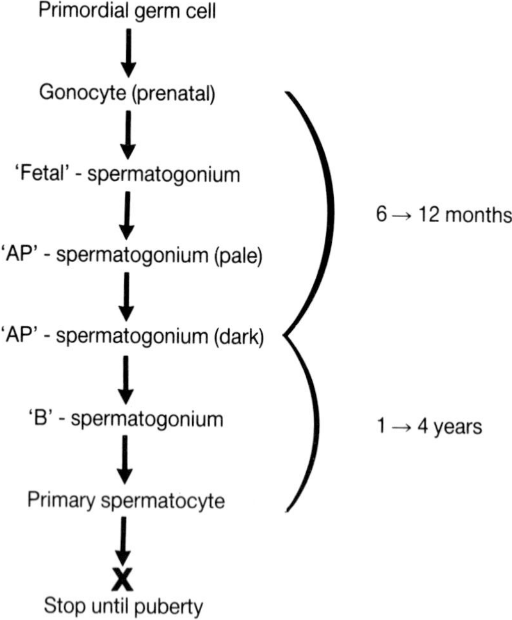

Figure 5.6 Schema showing the stages of germ cell maturation relative to age in humans.

Schindler *et al.*[35] reported the results of 441 biopsies from cryptorchid testes, in which germ cell counts were diminished in nearly all cases. Only 7 boys in this large group had normal germ cell populations, and 4 of these 7 boys were below 1 year of age. In a report of 257 testicular biopsies Saito and Kumamoto[36] found a significantly decreased ratio of germ cells per tubule in undescended testes, with the lowest ratios in the highest testes. In addition, normal histology was found in only 13 biopsies of 29 retractile testes. Decreased numbers of germ cells were also found in about 30% of the contralateral testes in unilateral cryptorchidism.

Using sophisticated histological techniques with plastic embedding of the testicular biopsies, Huff *et al.*[37] studied 232 biopsies from unilateral cryptorchid testes and 195 contralateral descended testes. Decreased numbers of germ cells were documented from the first year of life. The transformation of gonocytes to AD spermatogonia which normally is complete around 6 months of age was delayed or defective (Figure 5.6). In addition, the transformation of AD spermatogonia to primary spermatocytes which normally commences at about 3 years of age and is complete by about 4–5 years was also delayed or absent (Figure 5.7). They concluded that undescended testes showed features of

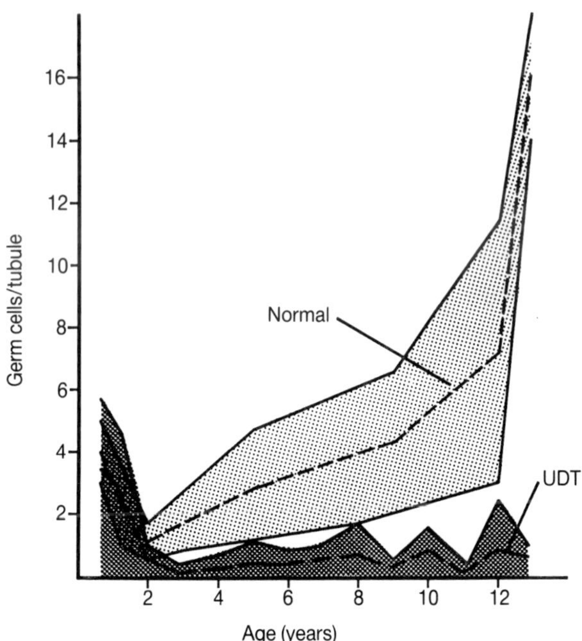

Figure 5.7 The mean number of germ cells per tubule in normal, compared with undescended testes (UDT). The standard deviation is indicated by the shaded areas. (Redrawn from Reference 37.)

hypogonadotrophic hypogonadism as the cause of the increased instance of infertility in these patients.

5.3.3 Compensatory testicular hypertrophy

A number of other morphological effects of undescended testes have been reported. Lauren *et al.*[38] reported compensatory testicular hypertrophy in the contralateral testes in 12% of children with unilateral undescended testes. They speculated that the frequency of contralateral hypertrophy would be greater except for the fact that the contralateral testis also appears to have undergone secondary dysplasia.

5.3.4 Testicular–epididymal fusion abnormalities

There are a number of reports of non-union between the testis and the epididymis in undescended testes.[39,40] This is a common associated abnormality when the gonad is located inside the canal or the abdomen (see Figures 4.15 (page 71) and 7.17 (page 134)). By contrast in testes which have descended through the external inguinal ring the incidence of epididymal abnormalities is about 10%. These abnormalities are thought to be related to underlying androgen deficiency *in utero,* although they have a significant effect on the subsequent outcome because they are not amenable to surgical correction.

5.4 Fertility

5.4.1 Fertility in the cryptorchid testis

Fertility in men with a history of cryptorchidism is significantly depressed, although this knowledge has been slow to accumulate. In the 1950s it was believed that there were no adverse changes in the undescended testes until after the advent of puberty. This led to the belief that surgical treatment was not necessary until 12–15 years of age.[42] It is now appreciated, as mentioned in the previous section, that germ cell maturation is already abnormal within the first year of life in boys with undescended testes.[33]

Fertility can be inhibited by cryptorchidism in animal experiments, where rats have been made surgically cryptorchid at birth.[43,42] Stewart and Brown[43] showed that germ cells were absent from the undescended testis and slightly deficient in the contralateral descended testis in adult life in rats so treated. Paternity rates, however, failed to reflect this dysfunction with the cryptorchid rats still having a 60% ability to produce offspring. Juenemann *et al.*[44] have shown in rat experiments that bilateral cryptorchidism causes suppression of fertility regardless of whether the undescended testes were produced mechanically by surgery or endocrinologically by oestrogen treatment postnatally.

Puri and O'Donnell[45] studied a cohort of 142 patients in Ireland, who had undergone orchidopexy at age 7–13½ years and found that fertility was related to the original position of the testes. The position of the testes had a variable effect on the sperm count, but most azospermic men had had canalicular or abdominal testes.

5.4.2 Fertility in the retractile testis

There is evidence that so-called retractile testes may lead to suppressed fertility later in life. Nistal and Paniagua[46] studied 23 infertile men whose only significant past history was bilateral retractile testes during childhood. These men showed oligospermia or azoospermia, and histological biopsies showed similar abnormalities to that seen in undescended testes. Rasmussen *et al.*[47] studied the fertility of 45 men who had apparent undescended testes during childhood but where the testes descended spontaneously at puberty. Only one third of these men had a normal semen analysis, and the majority had elevated levels of FSH consistent with impaired spermatogenesis. This study demonstrates that testes that may have been classified as 'high retractile' in the past and that descend spontaneously at puberty, have a significant morphological and functional abnormality in adult life that is similar to the abnormalities seen in true undescended testes.

In a study of 43 adults who as children had been diagnosed as having bilateral retractile testes, Puri and Nixon[48] found that 74% of the married patients had children, a rate that did not differ significantly from the general population. However, paternity was not established and semen was not analysed.

5.5 Malignancy

At one time it was believed that the incidence of neoplasia in men with previous history of cryptorchidism was 35–50 times greater than that of normal men.[49] This was based on a 10% frequency of a past history of cryptorchidism in men with testicular tumours compared with an expected incidence of undescended testes in the adult population of approximately 0.3% (as determined by statistics from army recruits). In recent years, however, it has been appreciated that the incidence of undescended testes in infancy approximates 1½–2% rather than 0.3%. This suggests that a more accurate figure for the relative risk of developing a testicular tumour in men with a history of cryptorchidism may be approximately 5–10 times that of the normal population.[50] In a detailed epidemiological study of 1116 men with testicular neoplasms in Victoria, Stone *et al.*[51] found an increased risk in those with a past history of cryptorchidism. They found a relative risk for men with unilateral undescended testis was 15, compared with 33 for bilateral undescended testes. The risk was seven times greater in the unilateral undescended testis, compared with the descended contralateral one. Seminomas were the most common tumours. A long-term review of 224 men treated as boys for cryptorchildism (at mean age 8 years) between 1935 and 1974 showed a standardized morbidity ratio of 11.4 (with 95% confidence intervals of 1.4 to 41.1). This study from the Mayo Clinic[52] shows a similar risk of cancer in USA as seen in UK[53] and Australia. Most authors agree with Stone *et al.*[51] that the risk of malignancy is much greater with intra-abdominal testes, compared with testes palpable in the groin.

The histological changes of progressive dysplasia observed in undescended testes are the putative cause of this increased risk of malignancy.[1,54,55] These tumours tend to occur at the same age as testicular tumours in normally descended testes, that is between 20 and 40 years of age. Fine-needle aspiration biopsies have been used recently to assess malignant change, and DNA flow cytometric analysis of these specimens does show aneuploidy in some men, suggestive of preneoplastic dysplasia.[56]

Secondary histological and functional abnormalities have been documented in the contralateral descended testis in males with unilateral undescended testis, and perhaps not surprisingly, therefore, 15–20% of all testicular tumours occur in the contralateral descended testis. Giwercman *et al.*[1] have speculated that the testicular tumours may be caused by an intrinsic abnormality in the testis which led to its initial maldescent, rather than to any secondary dysplasia caused by abnormally high temperature. In support of their theory, they suggest that carcinoma-*in-situ* germ cells (which they believe are the forerunner for invasive germ cell tumours) are in fact malignant gonocytes. Since germ cells that demonstrate histological characteristics of carcinoma-*in-situ* have been found in neonates with dysgenetic testes and ambiguous genitalia, these authors speculate that this is a primary rather than a secondary abnormality (Figure 5.8). The histological features of carcinoma-*in-situ* affecting the germ cells have been documented by Skakkabaek *et al.*[57] who have provided strong evidence that these abnormal cells are a prerequisite to invasive tumours of the testes. Giwercman *et al.*[58] followed up 500 men who had been admitted consecutively to a group of Danish hospitals with a previous diagnosis of testicular maldescent. Three hundred of these men consented to testicular biopsies where carcinoma-*in-situ* was diagnosed in five patients (1.7%). Abnormal germ cell development was found in two-thirds of the men. Because of their reported incidence of carcinoma-*in-situ* of approximately 2% they recommend that young adult males with a past history of undescended testes should be offered testicular biopsy to

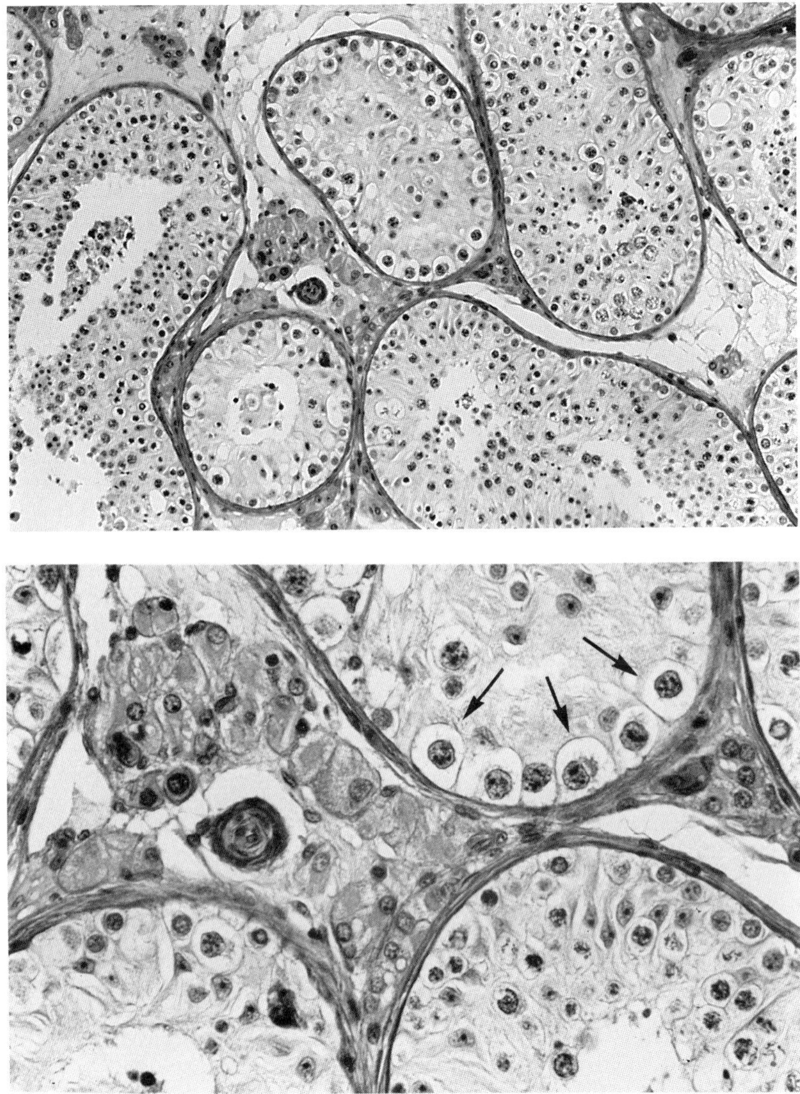

Figure 5.8 Histological pictures of the testis from an adult with carcinoma-*in-situ* and a past history of undescended testes (kindly provided by Prof N Skakkebaek). (a) Low-power view showing a normal seminiferous tubule on the right and a tubule with abnormal germ cells in the centre (×90). (b) High-power view showing carcinoma-*in-situ* germ cells (arrows) in one tubule adjacent to normal Leydig cells and normal tubules (×360).

exclude this condition before invasive tumour supervenes. Removal of the testis or irradiation appears curative.

References

1. Giwercman A, Muller J, Skakkebaek NE. Cryptorchidism and testicular neoplasia. *Hormone Res* 1988; **30:** 157–63.
2. Sutthoff-Lorey G, Waag KL. (1990). Die pra und intraoperative genebetemperaturmessung bei Maldescensus testis. In: Schier F, Waldschmidt J, eds. *Maldescensus Testis*. Munich: Zuckschwerdt Verlag, 1990: pp. 76–81.
3. Bedford JM. Anatomical evidence for the epididymis as the prime mover in the evolution of the scrotum. *Am J Anat* 1978; **152:** 483–508.
4. Steinberger A. Effects of temperature on the biochemistry of the testis. *Adv Exp Med Biol* 1991; **286:** 33–47.
5. Zorgniotti AA (ed). *Temperature and Environmental Effects on the Testis. Adv Exp Med Biol*. New York: Plenum Press, 1991: Vol. 286.
6. Grizard G, Azzaoui A, Boucher D. Testosterone, androstenedione, progesterone and 17α-hydroxyprogesterone in plasma and testes of immature rats under basal conditions and after hCG stimulation. Effect of bilateral cryptorchidism. *J Steroid Biochem* 1987; **28:** 703–10.
7. Farrer JH, Sikka SC, Xie HW, Constantinide D, Rajfer J. Impaired testosterone biosynthesis in cryptorchidism. *Fertil Steril* 1985; **44:** 125–32.
8. Huhtaniemi I, Bergh A, Nikula H, Damber J-E. Differences in the regulation of steroidogenesis and tropic hormone receptors between the scrotal and abdominal testes of unilaterally cryptorchid adult rats. *Endocrinology* 1984; **115:** 550–5.
9. Bergh A, Nikula H, Damber J-E, Clayton R, Huhtaniemi I. Altered concentrations of gonadotrophin, prolactin and GnRH receptors, and endogenous steroids in the abdominal testes of adult unilaterally cryptorchid rats. *J Reprod Fertil* 1985; **74:** 279–86.
10. Bergh A, Damber J-E, Ritzen M. Early signs of Sertoli and Leydig cell dysfunction in the abdominal testes of immature unilaterally cryptorchild rats. *Int J Androl* 1984; **7:** 398–408.
11. Abney TO, Keel BA (eds). *The Cryptotoid Testis*. Boca Raton, Florida: CRC Press, 1989.
12. Keel BA, Abney TO. Alterations of testicular function in the unilaterally cryporchid rat. *Proc Soc Exp Biol Med*. 1980; **116:** 489–95.
13. Keel BA, Abney TO. Influence of bilateral cryptorchidism in mature rat: alterations in testicular function and hormone levels. *Endocrinology* 1980; **107:** 1226–33.
14. Schanbacher BD, Grofjar HE jr. Keel BA. Testicular regulation of gonadotropin microheterogeneity: effects of cryptorchidism. In: *The Cryptorchid Testis* (Abney TO, Keel BA (eds). Boca Raton, Florida: CRC Press, 1989, pp 55–70.
15. de Kretser DM, Risbridger GP. Changes in sertoli cell structure and function. In: *The Cryptorchid Testis* (Abney TO, Keel BA eds). Boca Raton, Florida: CRC Press, 1989, pp 119–132.
16. Lee PA, Hoffman WH, White JJ, Engel RME, Blizzard RM. Serum gonadotropins in cryptorchidism. *Am J Dis Child* 1974; **127:** 530–2.
17. Koch H, Rahlf G. Endocrinologic and morphologic investigations in 208 prepubertal, pubertal or postpubertal patients with cryptorchidism. *Acta Endocrinol Suppl* 1975; 193 (85):85.
18. Walsh PC, Norvelle C, Mills RC, Siiteri PK. Plasma androgen response to hCG stimulation in prepubertal boys with hypospadias and cryptorchidism. *J Clin Endocrinol Metab* 1976; **42:** 52–9.

19. Waaler PE. Endocrinological studies in undescended testes. *Acta Paediatr Scand* 1976; **65:** 559–64.
20. Gendrel D, Roger M, Job J-C. Plasma gonadotropin and testosterone values in infants with cryptorchidism. *J Pediatr* 1980; **97:** 217–20.
21. Jockenhovel F, Swerdloff RS. Alterations in the steroidogenic capacity of Leydig cells in cryptorchid testis. In: Abney TO, Keel BA, eds. *The Cryptorchid Testis*. Boca Raton, Florida: CRC Press, 1989, pp. 35–54.
22. Van Vliet G, Caulfriez A, Robyn C, Wolter R. Plasma gonadotropin values in prepubertal cryptorchid boys: increase in FSH secretion in uni- and bilateral cases. *J Pediatr* 1980; **97:** 253–5.
23. Hovatta O, Huhtaniemi I, Wahlstrom T. Testicular gonadotrophins and their receptors in human cryptorchidism as revealed by immunohistochemistry and radioreceptor assay. *Acta Endocrinol* 1986; **111:** 128–32.
24. Baker BA, Morley R, Lucas A. Plasma testosterone in preterm infants with cryptorchidism. *Arch Dis Child* 1988; **63:** 1198–1200.
25. Job J-C, Toublanc J-E, Chaussain J-L, Gendrel D, Garnier P, Roger M. Endocrine and immunological findings in cryptorchid infants. *Hormone Res* 1988; **30:** 167–72.
26. Brown TR, Berkovitz GD, Gearheart JP. Androgen receptors in boys with isolated bilateral cryptorchidism. *Am J Dis Child* 1988; **142:** 933–6.
27. Baker M, Metcalfe SA, Hutson JM. Serum levels of MIS in boys from birth to 18 years, as determined by enzyme immunoassay. *J Clin Endocrinol Metab* 1990; **70:** 11–15.
28. Yamanaka J, Baker M, Metcalfe S, Hutson JM. Serum levels of Müllerian inhibiting substance in boys with cryptorchidism. *J Ped Surg* 1991; **26:** 621–3.
29. Scorer CG, Farrington GH. Congenital deformities of the testis and epididymis. London: Butterworths, 1971.
30. Mengel W, Hienz HA, Sippe WG, Hecker W Ch. Studies on cryptorchidism: a comparison of histological findings in the germinative epithelium before and after the second year of life. *J Pediatr Surg* 1974; **9:** 445–50.
31. Hadziselimovic F, Herzog B, Seguchi H. Surgical correction of cryptorchidism at 2 years: electron microscopic and morphometric investigations. *J Pediatr Surg* 1975; **10:** 19–26.
32. Hadziselimovic F, Herzog B, Girard J, Stalder G. Cryptorchidism – histology, fertility and treatment. *Prog Reprod Biol Med* 1984; **10:** 1–15.
33. Hadziselimovic F. Fertility and cryptorchidism. *Amer J Dis Child* 1985; **139:** 963–4.
34. Monet-Kuntz C, Barenton B, Locatelli A, Fontaine I, Perreau C, Hochereau-de Reviers MT. Effects of experimental cryptorchidism and subsequent orchidopexy on seminiferous tubule functions in the lamb. *J Androl* 1987; **8:** 148–54.
35. Schindler AM, Diaz P, Cuendet A, Sizonenko PC. Cryptorchidism: a morphological study of 670 biopies. *Helv Paediatr Acta* 1987; **42:** 45–158.
36. Saito S, Kumamoto Y. The number of spermatogonia in various congenital testicular disorders. *J Urol* 1989; **141:** 1166–8.
37. Huff DS, Hadziselimovic F, McC Snyder H, Duckett JW, Keating MA. Postnatal testicular maldevelopment in unilateral cryptorchidism. *J Urol* 1989; **142:** 546–8.
38. Lauren Z, Dickerman Z, Ritterman I. Compensatory testicular hypertrophy in unilateral cryptorchidism. *Pediatr Adolesc Endocrinol* 1979; **6:** 137–47.
39. Johansen TEB. Anatomy of the testis and epididymis in cryptorchidism. *Andrologia* 1987; **19:** 565–9.
40. Johansen TEB. Non-union of testis and epididymis. *Scand J Urol Nephrol* 1988; **22:** 165–70.

41. Nelson WO. Some problems of testicular function. *J Urol* 1953; **69:** 325–38.
42. Kogan BA, Gupta R, Juenemann K-P. Fertility in cryptorchidism: further development of an experimental model. *J Urol* 1987; **137:** 128–31.
43. Stewart RJ, Brown S. Fertility in experimental unilateral cryptorchidism. *J Pediatr Surg* 1990; **25:** 672–4.
44. Juenemann K-P, Kogan BA, Abozeid MH. Fertility in cryptorchidism: an experimental model. *J Urol* 1986; **136:** 214–8.
45. Puri P, O'Donnell B. Semen analysis of patients who had orchidopexy at or after seven years of age. *Lancet* 1988; **ii:** 1051–2.
46. Nistal M, Paniagua R. Infertility in adult males with retractile testes. *Fertil Steril* 1984; **41:** 395–403.
47. Rasmussen BT, Ingerslev HJ, Hostrup H. Bilateral spontaneous descent of the testis after the age of 10: subsequent effects on fertility. *Br J Surg* 1988; **75:** 820–3.
48. Puri P, Nixon HH. Bilateral retractile testes – subsequent effects on fertility. *J Pediatr Surg* **12:** 563–7.
49. Whitaker RH. Neoplasia in cryptorchid men. *Semin Urol* 1988; **6:** 107–9.
50. Woodhouse CRJ. Undescended testes. In: *Long-term Paediatric Urology*. Oxford: Blackwell Scientific. 1991.
51. Stone JM, Cruickshank DG, Sandeman TF, Matthews JP. Laterality, maldescent, trauma and other clinical factors in the epidemiology of testis cancer in Victoria, Australia. *Br J Cancer* 1991; **64:** 132–8.
52. Benson RC, Beard CM, Kelalis PP, Kurland LT. Malignant potential of the cryptorchid testis. *Mayo Clin Proc* 1991; **66:** 372–8.
53. Chilvers C, Pike MC. Epidemiology of undescended testis. In: Oliver RTD, Blandy JP, Hopestone HF, eds. *Urological and Genital Cancer*. Oxford: Blackwell Scientific, 1989: pp. 306–21.
54. Campbell HE. The incidence of malignant growth of the undescended testicle: a reply and re-evaluation. *J Urol* 1959; **81:** 663–8.
55. Haughey BP, Graham S, Brasure J, Zielezny M, Sufria G, Burnett WS. The epidemiology of testicular cancer in upstate New York. *Am J Epidemiol* 1989; **130:** 25–36.
56. Clausen OPF, Giwercman A, Jorgensen N, Bruun E, Frimodt-Moller C, Skakkebaek NE. DNA distribution in maldescensus testes: hyperdiploid aneuploidy without evidence of germ cell neoplasia. *Cytometry* 1991; **12:** 77–81.
57. Skakkebaek NE, Berthelsen JG, Giwercman A, Muller J. Carcinoma in situ of the testis: possible origin from gonocytes and precursor of all types of germ cell tumors except spermatocytomas. *Int J Androl* 1987; **10:** 19–28.
58. Giwercman A, Bruun E, Frimodt-Moller CAI, Skakkebaek NS. Prevalence of carcinoma-*in-situ* and other histopathological abnormalities in testes of men with a history of cryptorchidism. *J Urol* 1989; **142:** 998–1002.

6

Diagnosis of undescended testis

6.1 Introduction

The clinical diagnosis of undescended testes in competent hands usually is straightforward. However, the number of children referred to paediatric surgical clinics with normal (but retractile) testes which could not be located by the primary referring practitioner, or who present in late childhood (or at infertility clinics as adults) with previously unrecognized cryptorchidism, testifies to the difficulties of making a correct diagnosis. This chapter describes the technique of examination and the methods available for the investigation of the common undescended and uncommon impalpable testis.

6.2 Aims of clinical examination

The purposes of clinical examination are (1) to identify the presence of a testis, and (2) to determine the lowest position in the line of normal descent that it can achieve. All testes have a range of movement and it is the lowest limit of this range, without tension on the spermatic cord, which is relevant. The lowest limit of the testicular position probably corresponds with the caudal limit of the processus vaginalis.

6.3 Technique of examination

The examination should be conducted in warm surroundings with the child relaxed. He should lie on a comfortable examination couch which is at a height that is comfortable for the clinican. When his clothing is removed to expose the genitalia, the appearance of the scrotum and any swellings in the inguinal region are noted. The position of the testes is then confirmed by palpation.

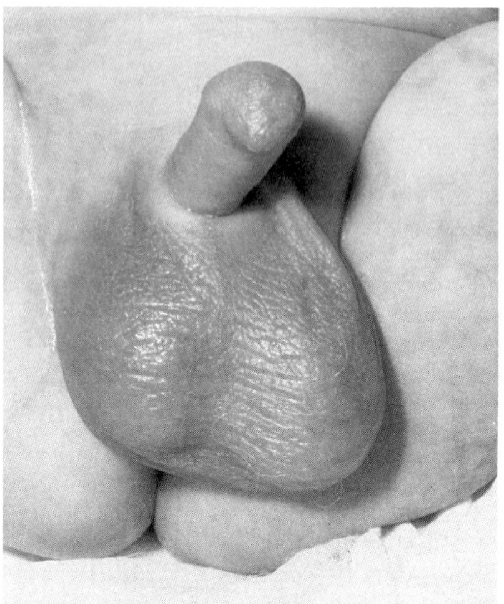

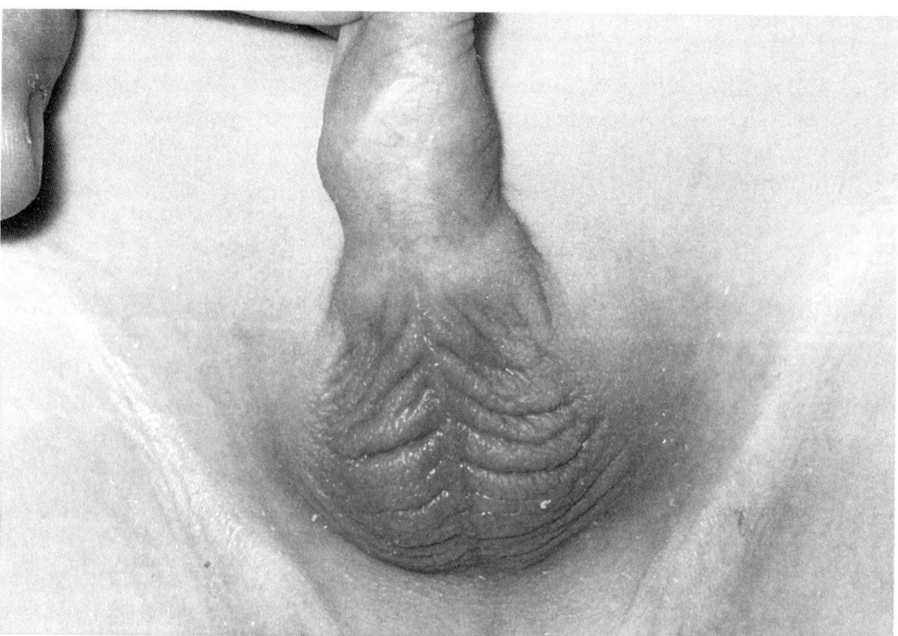

Figure 6.1 The appearance of the scrotum at different ages: (a) the thin, redundant and large scrotum of the neonate; and (b) the small puckered-up scrotum of middle childhood.

6.3.1 The appearance of the scrotum

There is considerable variation in the appearance of the scrotum at different ages and body types (Figure 6.1) When a testis is obviously in the scrotum at the commencement of examination, its exact location should be noted: whether it is at the bottom, the mid-scrotum or top (and subsequently whether it retracts out of it).

If two testes are seen lying spontaneously low in the scrotum, cryptorchidism is not present (Figure 6.2) An empty hemiscrotum is suggestive of either an undescended testis, retractile testis or absent testis.

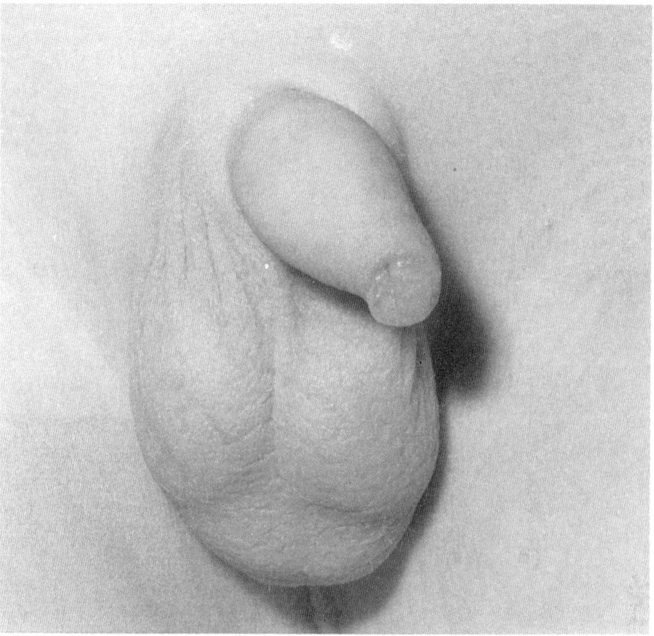

Figure 6.2 Normally descended testes readily seen lying in the scrotum of an 8-year-old boy.

When there is a retractile testis, the scrotum is usually well developed and similar to the contralateral side. An empty hemiscrotum of reasonable size suggests that the examiner could expect to bring a testis down into it, i.e. a retractile testis is likely (Figure 6.3).[1] A flat, small hemiscrotum is less likely to have had a testis residing in it (Figure 6.4) but is not diagnostic of cryptorchidism.

6.3.2 Location of the testis

When one or both halves of the scrotum are empty, the position of the testis(es) should be determined. In Figure 6.4, one testis is fully descended,

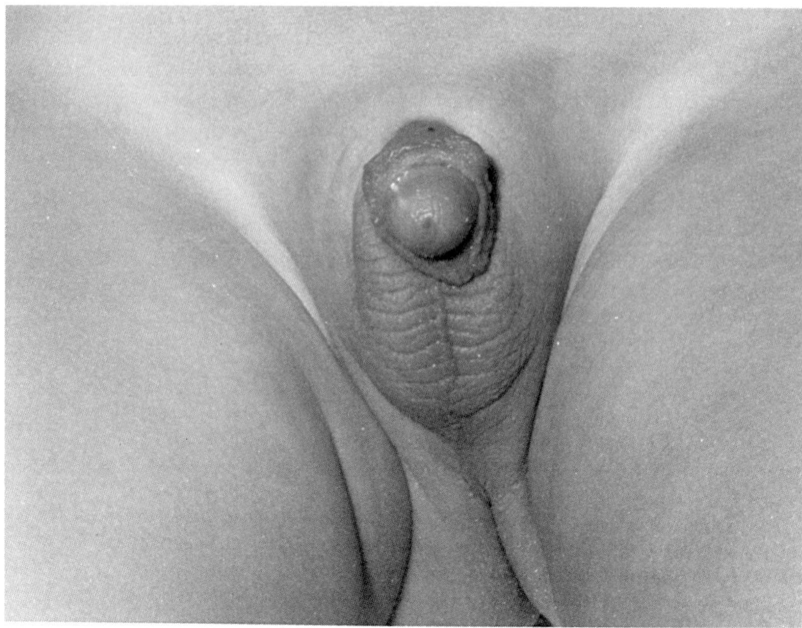

Figure 6.3 Where there is a unilateral retractile testis, both sides of the scrotum are of the same size.

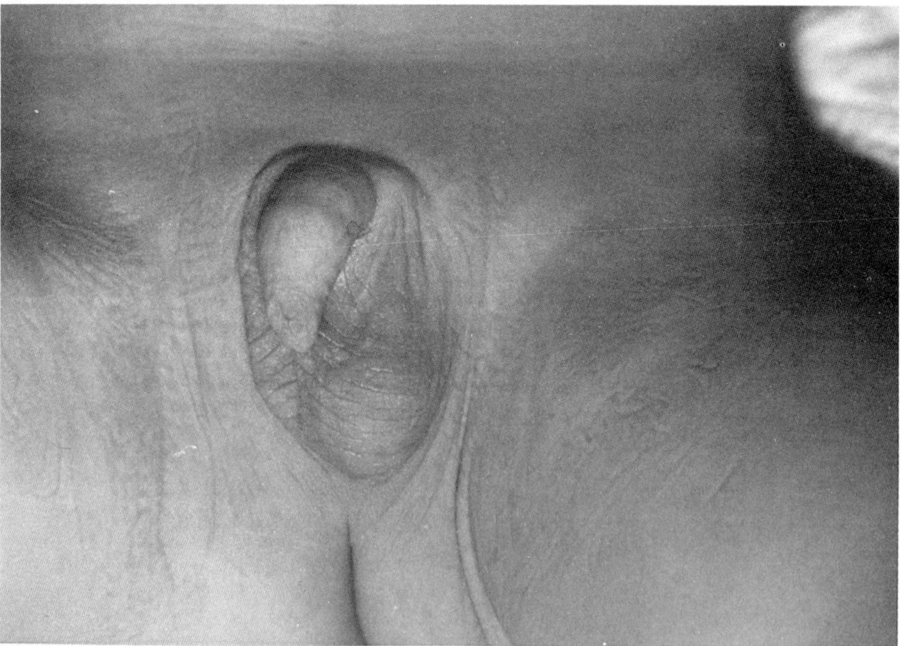

Figure 6.4 A flat small hemiscrotum suggests that a testis does not normally reside in it. In this child, the right testis is undescended.

whereas the other is out of the scrotum. When a testis is not evident in the scrotum, it is probably lying in the superficial inguinal pouch, lateral and superior to the pubic tubercle (see Chapter 4). It can best be felt with the flat of the fingers of one hand which milk it downwards and medially along the line of the inguinal canal towards the scrotum (Figure 6.5).

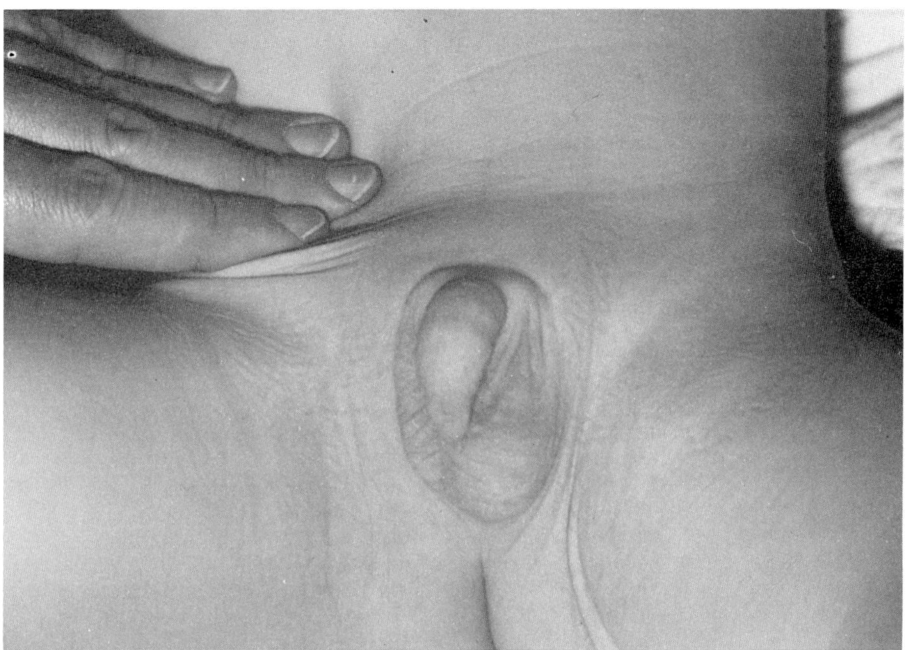

Figure 6.5 The undescended right testis lying in the superficial inguinal pouch can best be felt with the flat of the fingers of the hand which 'milks' it downwards and medially along the line of the inguinal canal towards the scrotum.

While the testis is being moved over the pubis, the thumb and index finger of the other hand can grasp it through the scrotal skin to assess the lowest level to which it can be manipulated (Figure 6.6) In this way, the testis is brought (if possible) into the scrotum and its exact and lowest position noted. If tension on the cord prevents the testis reaching the bottom of the scrotum, the testis is undescended. It is also undescended if it can be pulled to the bottom of the scrotum under tension, but disappears as soon as it is released (Figure 6.7). If the testis can be released in the scrotum yet remains there for a short period before the cremasteric reflex returns it to the superficial pouch, it is described as being descended but retractile. Once a retractile (but descended) testis has been brought into the scrotum in this way, it can be released and observed, still within the scrotum, by drawing back the fingers overlying the pubic tubercle.

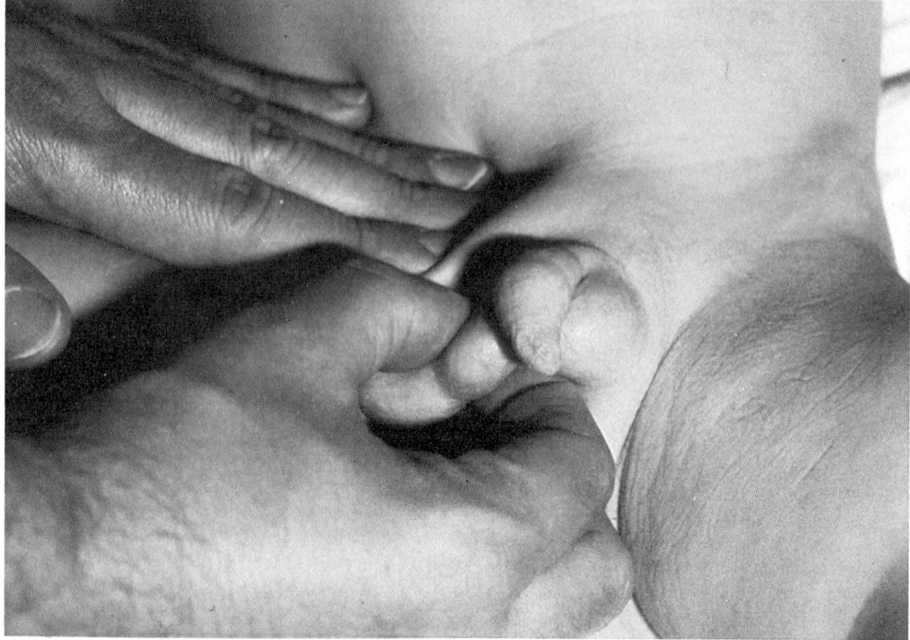

Figure 6.6 When the testis is coerced over the pubis, the thumb and index finger of the other hand can grasp it through the scrotal skin to assess the lowest level to which it can be manipulated.

An undescended testis may be impalpable initially, and only appear when it is 'milked' out of the inguinal canal (where it is concealed from detection by the overlying external oblique aponeurosis) to emerge at the external ring at which level it becomes palpable (and hence detectable clinically). This is sometimes referred to as an 'emergent testis'.

6.3.3 Description of the level of the testis

There are two main methods by which the positions of testes have been classified. The first was popularized by Scorer[2] who described a testis as being cryptorchid if the centre of the testis was less than 4 cm below the pubic tubercle, and 2.5 cm at the birth examination for babies weighing under 2500 g. All measurements were rounded down to the nearest 0.5 cm. Measurement is made after the testis is manipulated into its lowest position along the pathway of normal anatomical descent, without undue tension being applied to it (Figure 6.8). Application of these criteria defines an 'undescended testis by measurement'.[3] This method of documentation requires considerable precision.

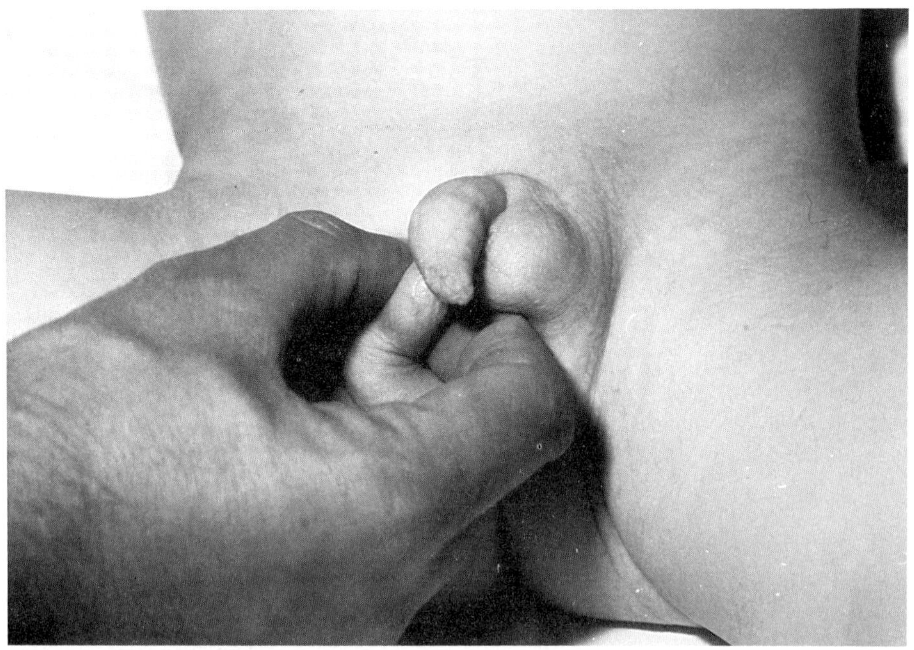

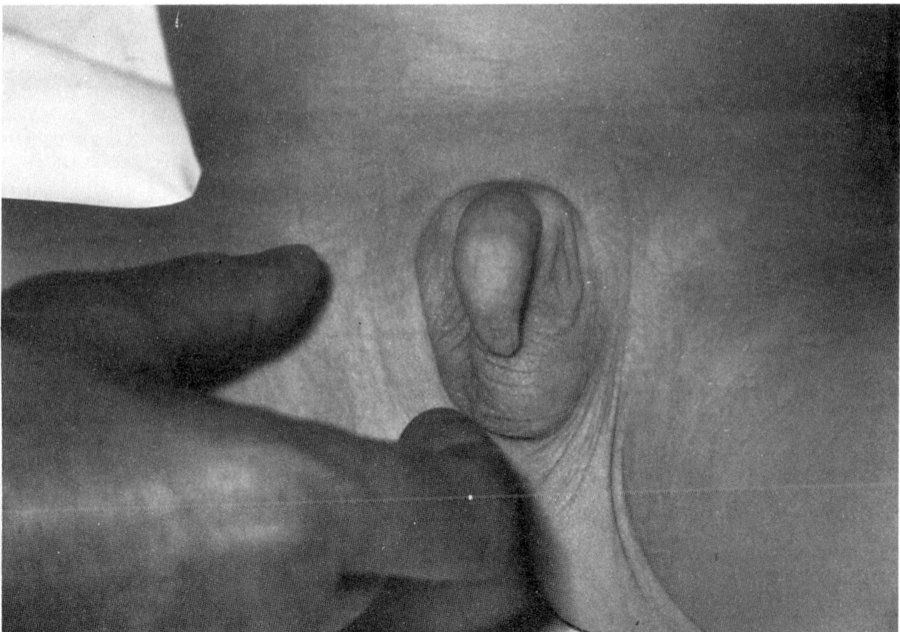

Figure 6.7 As soon as the true undescended testis is released it disappears from the scrotum. This is the same patient as in Figures 6.4–6.6

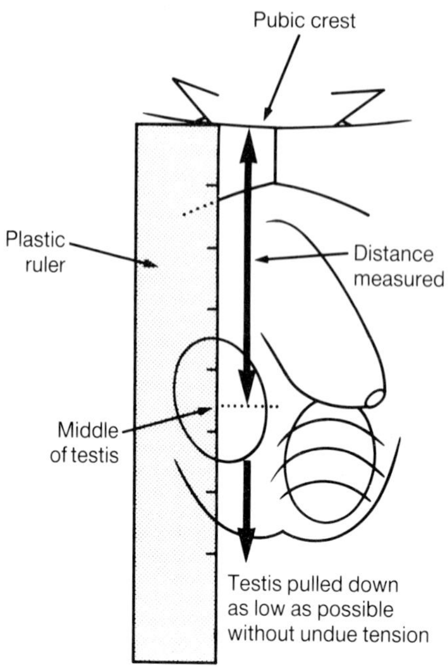

Figure 6.8 Measurement of the distance of descent from the pubic tubercle. The distance can be measured with a plastic ruler.

The second, and perhaps the more popular, method is to define the 'undescended testis by position.'[4] The position of each testis is classified as being: normal (well down in the scrotum); high scrotal; supra-scrotal (palpable, and in line of normal descent including the superficial inguinal pouch, but not in the scrotum – see Chapter 4); non-palpable; and 'other.' 'Other' includes ectopic; neonatal orchidopexy before examination; and position obscured by a hernia or hydrocele. This system classifies all testes which are not well down in the scrotum as being undescended. This method has a close correlation with that described by Scorer.

6.3.4 Examination in the newborn

Scorer[2] observed that the lower the birthweight, the higher the incidence of cryptorchidism. This applies even when premature babies are examined 3 months after their expected delivery date, rather than according to their chronological age, thus correcting for effects of low gestation by allowing extra time for the testes to descend spontaneously.[4]

The effective gestational age is an important factor in addition to that of birthweight. The Oxford study showed that testes of cryptorchid babies of less than 37 weeks' gestation are more likely to descend by the age of 3 months than in babies of longer gestation. The lower the testis is along the path of normal descent at birth, the higher the chance that the testis will descend spontaneously by 3 months of age.[4] The John Radcliffe study found that testes at the level of the pubic tubercle (i.e. zero measurement) have half the chance of spontaneous descent of those that are definitely below the pubic tubercle. The latter group is as likely to descend as the high scrotal testis.

The majority of boys born at full term have both testes fully descended in a large thin-walled scrotum. Testes are easily palpable and readily reach the bottom of the scrotum, which is proportionately much larger than later in childhood (see Figure 6.1a). On measurement, the testes are usually found 4–7 cm below the pubic crest.[5]

When a testis is not fully descended at birth, some descent may continue for several weeks following birth. Where no testis can be felt at birth, it is unlikely that full descent will still occur (except in the extremely premature). Descent ceases altogether at about 3 months of age. Therefore, repeated examination of infants in the first 3 months of life may give an accurate idea of where the undescended testis is ultimately going to lie, i.e. the lowest level to which it will descend.[5] There is no evidence that significant descent of the testis occurs in a full-term infant beyond 3–4 months of age. In a study of 3534 boys,[4] 210 (5.9%) were cryptorchid by measurement and 220 (6.2%) by position at birth. By 3 months of age, the rate of cryptorchidism was identical (1.6%) in both groups.

6.3.5 Examination of the premature infant

Because inguinoscrotal descent of the testis occurs in the seventh month of gestation, infants born at this time will often demonstrate undescended testes (Figure 6.9). The position and movement of the testes in these infants is easy to determine because the testis is relatively large at a time when there is little subcutaneous fat and the scrotum is undeveloped and relatively small compared with the full-term baby. The great majority of testes in these infants descend normally, and descent will be complete by term. There is also a higher incidence of inguinal herniae (see Section 6.3.6). If a testis is still undescended at 3 months post-term, it will remain so. As in full-term infants, the left testis is more commonly affected than the right.

6.3.6 Mobility of the testis

The great mobility of the testis within, and out of, the scrotum is permitted: (1) because the testis has no direct attachment to the scrotum; and (2) by virtue of patency of the processus vaginalis.[6] This non-adherence to the scrotum can be demonstrated by locating a fully descended testis in

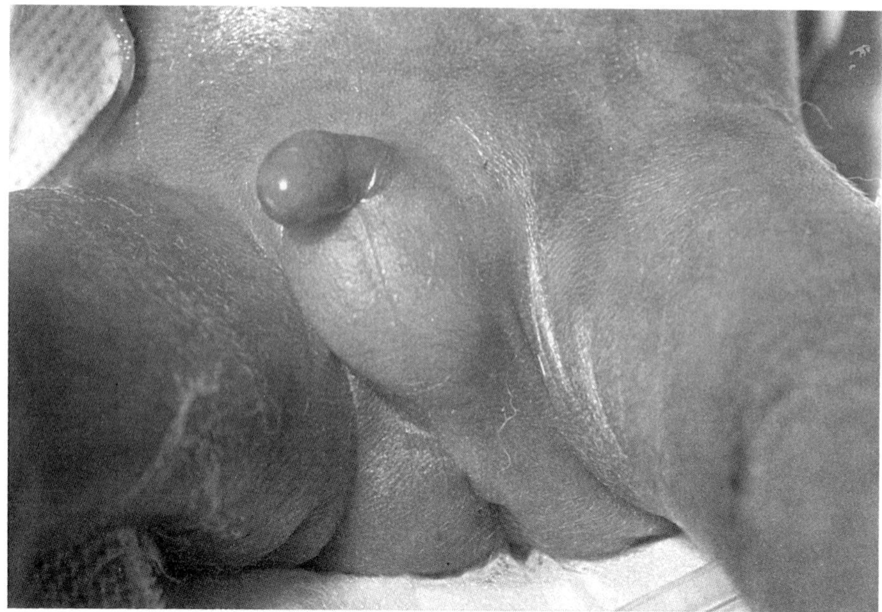

Figure 6.9 Undescended testes are often seen in premature infants born before 32 weeks' gestation. (Photo kindly provided by Dr Peter Morris.)

the scrotum and then displacing it upwards into the groin without any evidence of retraction or inversion of the scrotal skin (Figure 6.10). If, however, the testis is displaced even further from the scrotum (and distal attachment of the gubernaculum) inversion at the site of gubernacular attachment occurs: in a normally descended testis, this is in the scrotum; in an undescended testis, the attachment will be above the neck of the scrotum (Figure 6.11).

6.3.7 Cryptorchidism associated with a symptomatic hernia

Normally, the patent processus vaginalis begins to close proximally once the testis has reached the scrotum – and its lack of contents after the testis has descended probably assists in its contraction and ultimate obliteration. In the premature infant in particular, the testis is still occupying the processus, holding it open, and with the effect of peaks in intra-abdominal pressure (e.g. crying) herniation of bowel through the internal ring is more likely to occur. This may explain in part the apparent increased frequency of symptomatic herniae in the premature infant.

Occasionally, a strangulated inguinal hernia may occur in an infant who has an undescended testis (Figure 6.12). The infant presents with a tender, irreducible lump at the external ring, and the ipsilateral scrotum is

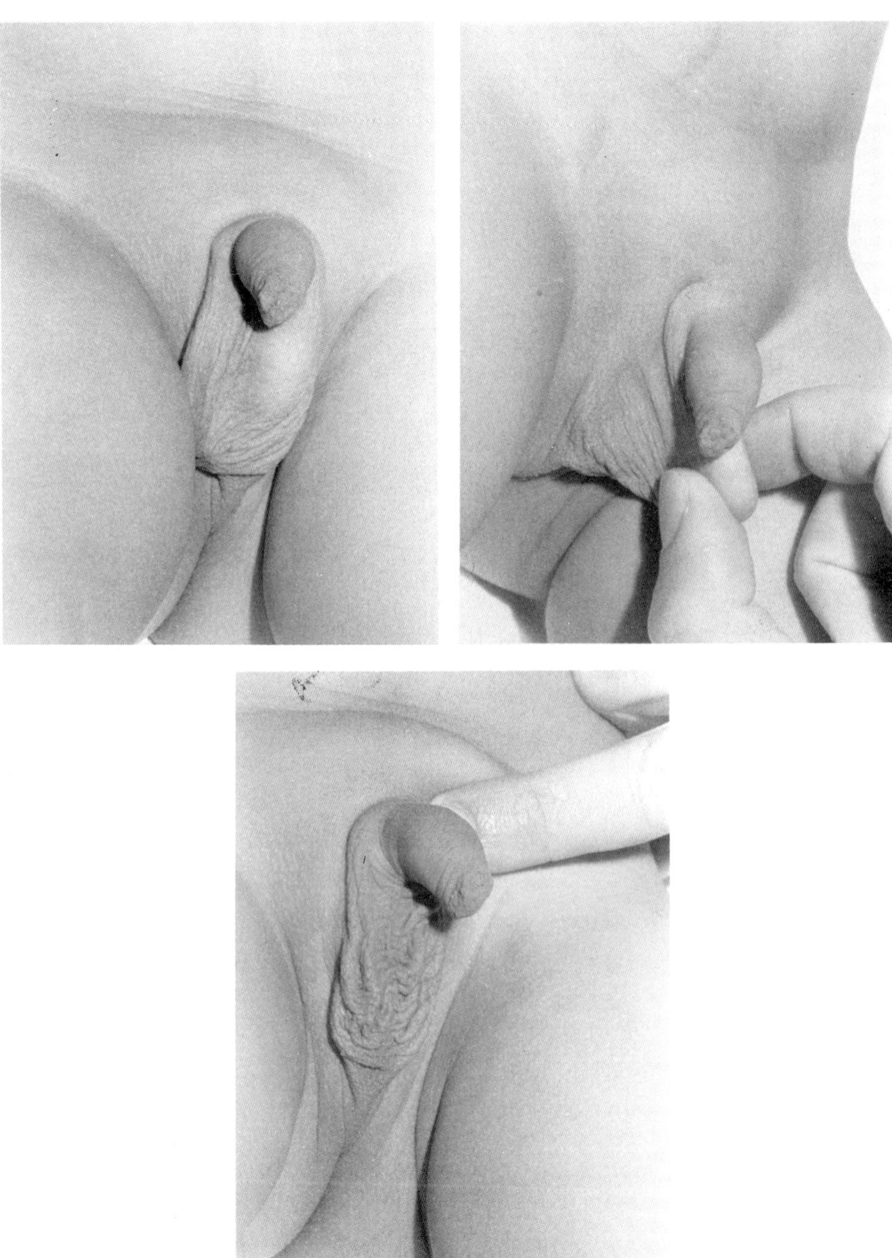

Figure 6.10 The mobility of the testis and its non-adherence to the scrotum. (a) This patient has a normally descended left testis. (b) The examining fingers can draw the testis well down into the scrotum and (c) displace it upwards out of the scrotum and into the groin without evidence of retraction or inversion of the scrotal skin. Note the undescended right testis.

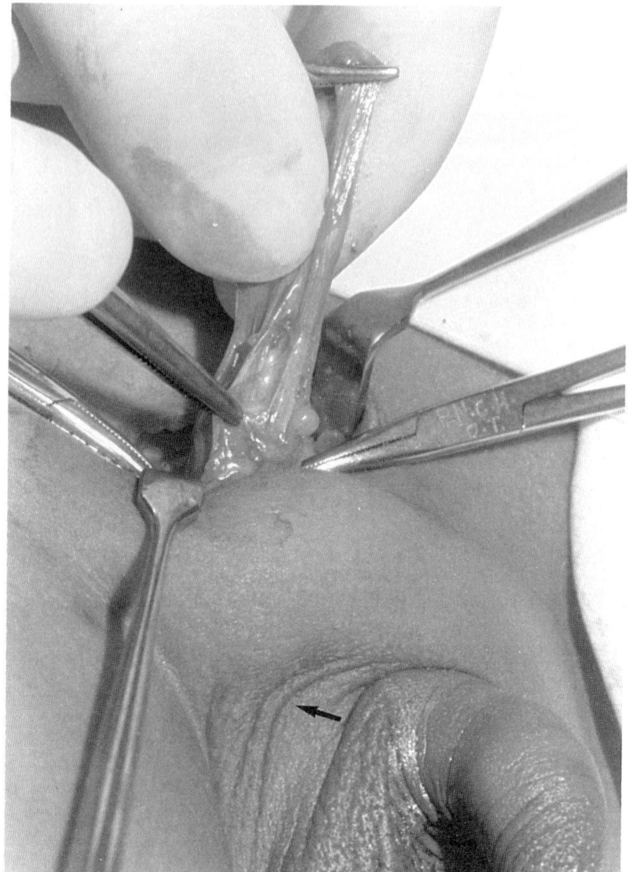

Figure 6.11 Traction on the gubernaculum of an undescended testis during orchidopexy causes the skin proximal to the neck of the scrotum to retract. *Black arrow:* puckering of the skin adjacent to the scrotum.

empty. Careful examination will reveal two components to the lump, one being the testis, the other the contents of the hernial sac. Gentle manipulation of the hernial component usually achieves its reduction, and at subsequent surgery orchidopexy is performed at the time of herniotomy. Failure to site the testis in the correct position in the scrotum at this time creates major technical problems later, since adhesions and scar tissue in the region of the internal inguinal ring make a later orchidopexy difficult.

A long-standing or tightly strangulated inguinal hernia can interfere with the blood supply to the testis. This may be evident at the time of herniotomy and orchidopexy, e.g. blood-stained fluid around the testis, or on review later, when the testis atrophies and disappears. Injury to the

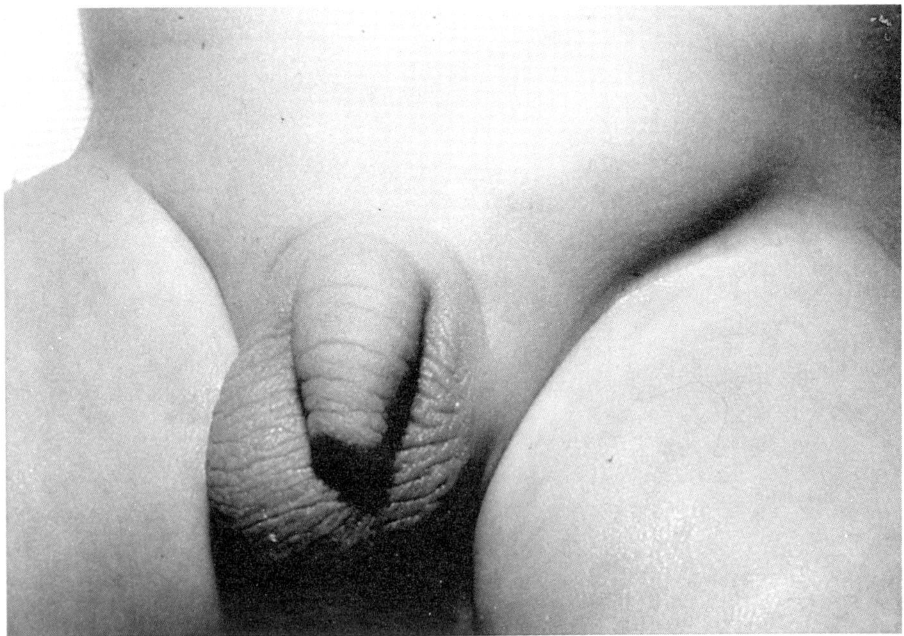

Figure 6.12 A strangulated left inguinal hernia in an infant with an undescended testis on one side and a hydrocele on the other.

testicular vessels during the operative procedure may also cause testicular atrophy, a reason that this procedure is best performed by a paediatric surgeon, whose expertise and familiarity with the region in infants makes inadvertent injury to the vascular supply of the testis less likely.

6.3.8 Apparent cryptorchidism with testicular torsion

Testicular torsion usually occurs during adolescence in boys with fully descended testes: only rarely are undescended testes involved. However, when the mesorchium of the testis, in which is contained the testicular vessels and vas deferens, twists, it lifts the testis up towards the neck of the scrotum which might give a false impression of the testis being 'high' to start with (Figure 6.13). It is almost certain that the testis was descended fully prior to the torsion.

6.4 Undescended testis versus retractile testis

An undescended testis must be distinguished clinically from a retractile testis. A true undescended testis cannot be manipulated to the bottom

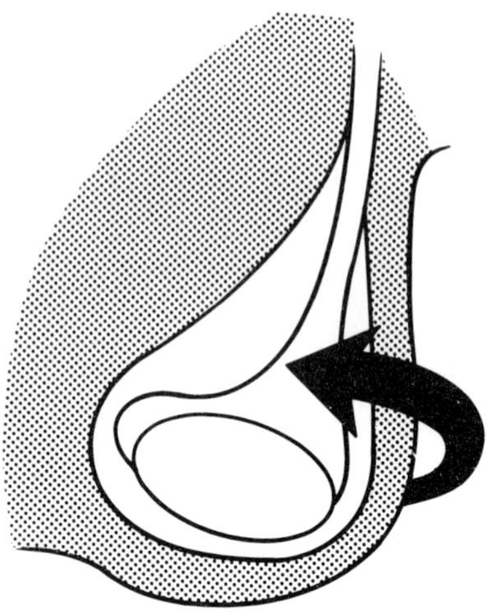

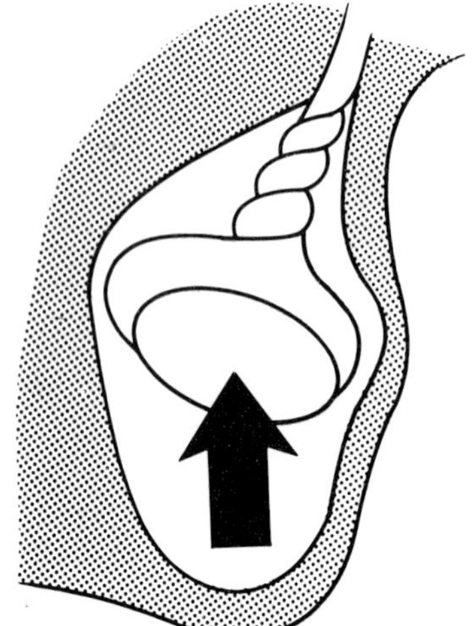

Figure 6.13 A testis undergoing torsion is usually suspended on a long mesorchium, which shortens during the process of twisting, resulting in the testis assuming an apparently higher position in the scrotum.

of the scrotum and remain there: even if it can be coerced into the upper scrotum further traction on it causes pain (from stretching of the spermatic cord) and as soon as it is released it adopts its original position out of the scrotum. On the other hand, a retractile testis is one that may be found initially outside the scrotum but can be brought down into a normal position in the scrotum, a reflection of the normal range of movement the child's testis is allowed. After manipulation into the scrotum, the testis stays there until the cremasteric reflex is stimulated.[6]

In most normal boys, the testes are always at the bottom of the scrotum; the cremasteric reflex produces a small upward movement, although the testes do not normally leave the scrotum.[1] There are many boys in whom one testis is stable at the bottom of the scrotum and one retracts. It is suspected that many retractile testes become higher as age increases, the so-called 'ascending testis'.[1,7,8] Thus it is important to consider the age of the child in relation to the position of the testis in the scrotum.

The main characteristics of a retractile testis may be summarized as follows:

(1) Can be brought fully to the bottom of the scrotum.
(2) Remains in the scrotum for a period before retracting. (Retraction is immediate if the cord is tight and the testis undescended.)
(3) The testis resides spontaneously in the scrotum at times.
(4) The testis is a normal size.

Two other features which may be useful in distinguishing retractile from undescended testes are:

(1) Testicular size. If the testis in question is smaller than an opposite 'normal' testis, retarded development (i.e. dysplasia) because of incomplete descent is likely.
(2) A normal testis can be held between the finger and thumb and traction exerted on the cord without causing pain. When the cord is abnormally tight, this manoeuvre causes pain at the lateral end of the inguinal canal, the site of the lateral suspensory fibres found at orchidopexy.[1]

The difficulty distinguishing a retractile from an undescended testis has prompted some clinicians to use human chorionic gonadotrophin (hCG). The rationale for treatment is that in cases of testicular retractility, hCG would be expected to induce testicular descent because testosterone has been produced.[9] Failure of hCG to achieve descent (and inhibit retractility) would suggest the testis is truly undescended.[10]

6.5 Clinical features of ectopic testes

6.5.1 Definition

When a testis migrates away from the normal pathway of descent to end up beyond the range of normal movement of the testis, it is said to be ectopic. It may occupy one of a wide variety of positions in the inguino-perineal region, as follows:

(1) Perineal testis.
(2) Pubo-penile testis.
(3) Femoral testis.
(4) Crossed-testicular ectopia.
(5) Exstrophy of the testis.
(6) Ectopia of the scrotum.

An ectopic testis may have a normal length of spermatic cord and simply require relocation in the scrotum. By the definition provided above, a testis in the superficial inguinal pouch is not considered ectopic (see Chapter 4).

6.5.2. Perineal testis

The infant presents with an empty hemiscrotum and an adjacent perineal swelling (see Figure 4.3, page 54). If unrecognized at birth, it may present later in life with perineal pain following sitting in certain positions or during sexual excitation.[11] The swelling is behind the scrotum but anterior to the anus and to one side of the median raphe.[5] The long axis of the testis is directed anteroposteriorly. There is usually a normally descended testis on the other side: bilateral cases are rare,[12] but occasionally there may be an undescended testis on the other side.[13] The perineal testis is well developed and normal in size, and the epididymis has a normal relationship to the testis. Microscopic studies[14,15] suggest histological changes similar to that seen in true undescended testes. It is likely that, although the pre-pubertal perineal testis could be considered 'normal', if untreated, secondary degenerative changes may occur.

The spermatic cord of the perineal testis is of ample length,[11] which allows for easy mobilization into the scrotum during orchidopexy.

6.5.3 Pubo-penile testis

In this rare condition, the testis is found to lie subcutaneously on the dorsal aspect of the penis near its base, close to the pubic bone.[5]

6.5.4 Femoral testis

A femoral location is a rare place for an ectopic testis. Usually it has descended through the inguinal canal but then migrated infero-laterally into the subcutaneous tissue of the thigh. However, descent of the testis through the femoral canal has been reported on rare occasions.[16,17] The lower end of the gubernaculum appears to occupy the femoral ring, rather than protruding through the external inguinal ring. One would expect that descent should only take place into the subcutaneous tissues of the thigh, but in two cases[17,18] the testis still managed to reach the scrotum.

6.5.5. Inguino-perineal testis

The inguino-perineal ectopic testis may be found initially in the superficial inguinal space but cannot be manipulated into the scrotum. Instead, it passes lateral to the scrotum. In other boys it may be identified residing spontaneously lateral to the scrotum in the medial aspect of the upper thigh or even beyond the scrotum (Figure 6.14).

6.5.6 Crossed testicular ectopia

In this rare condition one testis descends (usually incompletely) down the contralateral processus vaginalis.[19] It has been discussed more fully in Chapter 4.

6.5.7 Testicular exstrophy

In this extremely rare condition, the testis is exposed through a defect in the skin of the neck of the scrotum.[20,21] A potential explanation for this

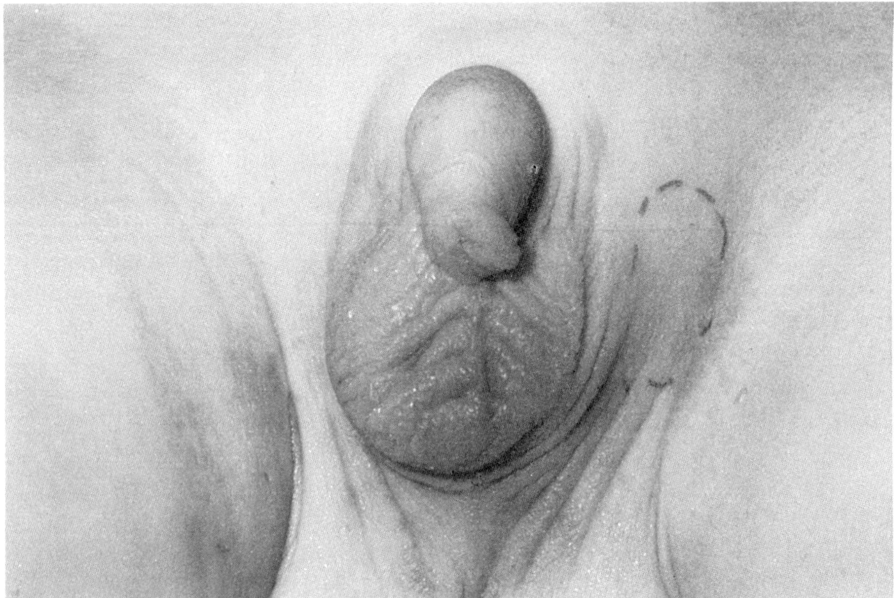

Figure 6.14 An inguino-perineal ectopic testis lying lateral to the scrotum.

anomaly proposed by FD Stephens (personal communication) is that there is local compression of the scrotum by the heel of the fetus, leading to skin necrosis, with secondary prolapse of the testis through the defect.

6.5.8 Ectopia of the scrotum

In these rare infants, the testis descends normally into the scrotum but the scrotum itself is ectopic.[22,23] Abnormalities of the genito-urinary and skeletal systems are common associations of this bizarre defect.

6.6 Impalpable testis

6.6.1 Purpose of investigation

Nearly all undescended testes have migrated at least as far as the external inguinal ring. If a testis is impalpable when examined by an experienced paediatric clinician (usually a paediatric surgeon) it means that it is either: (a) absent; or (b) intracanalicular or intra-abdominal.

If a testis is present it should be identified because of the risk of malignancy[24] and because of the potential for sterility.

6.6.2 Clinical examination

Many apparently 'impalpable' testes, when the child is examined by a primary medical practitioner, can be palpated by a paediatric surgeon. This is most likely to occur in an older child who has markedly retractile testes, or who is obese, where the testis was not detected in the groin because of its mobility or the thick layer of subcutaneous fat. Every effort should be made to coerce a potentially intracanalicular testis through the external ring, as described earlier in this chapter. Failure to achieve this will necessitate performance of one or more of the investigations summarized below:

(1) Imaging techniques:
   (a) Ultrasound.
   (b) CT scan.
   (c) Magnetic resonance imaging.
   (d) Selective renography.
   (e) Arteriography.
(2) Laparoscopy.
(3) Surgical exploration.

Infants and small children with bilateral impalpable testes should have an hCG stimulation test[25] to confirm that functional testicular tissue is present. When the immunoassay for müllerian inhibiting substance becomes available for clinical work, it is likely to supplant the hCG-stimulation test since it requires only one blood sample (see Chapter 5).

6.6.3 Ultrasonography

Ultrasound is a non-invasive technique which has been used to identify impalpable testes. Early reports suggested that ultrasonography was reasonably successful in the search for intracanalicular testes but was of less value for the intra-abdominal testis. For example, Madrazo *et al.*[26] were unable to find intra-abdominal testes, whereas they identified 8 of 9 intracanalicular testes. Other authors have also questioned the reliability of the technique[27] when used to locate intra-abdominal testes.

In a more recent report of 60 examinations, the sonographic results agreed with the surgical findings in 88%.[28] Transducer frequencies of 5–7.5 mHz were used, and mHz information was easier to interpret using a static B-scanner because of its ability to include a larger area of interest within the same scan. However, it appears that there was only one intra-abdominal testis (and four absent testes), and they acknowledged that interference from adjacent structures made localization of testes on the abdominal side of the internal ring impossible. Hederstrom *et al.*[28] also cautioned that the infantile testis is not easily detectable and has a sonographic appearance which may be consistent with other structures – a further limiting factor in the applicability of the technique. The similarity in appearance with gubernacular structures may lead to false positive examinations.[29]

In one study[30] it is claimed that three intra-abdominal testes were identified on ultrasound but that they were all clinically palpable. Given the impalpability of abdominal testes and their definition of 'intra-abdominal' on ultrasound (anterior or lateral to the external iliac vessels) their description may merely have highlighted the problem of having few reliable landmarks in the localisation of the gonads using this technique.

The inguinal testis, for which an ultrasound may be an effective diagnostic tool, will be located easily during surgical exploration of the groin, making ultrasonography an unnecessary exercise.[31] Ultrasonography is not appropriate as a routine procedure for the evaluation of the undescended testis,[29] and has a very limited role in the examination of a child with an impalpable testis.

6.6.4 CT scan

Proponents of CT localization of the impalpable cryptorchid testis claim that the procedure is quick, simple, non-invasive and can be performed at all ages.[32,33] One disadvantage is the radiation required, and the necessity for intravenous contrast injection to distinguish major vessels from undescended testes in some patients.

The technique described by Wolverson *et al.*[32] involves scans at 125 kV and 60 mAs from the scrotum to anterosuperior iliac spines at 8 mm intervals and a scan time of 4 seconds. In children, detail of intra-abdominal structures is poor above this level because of the sparsity of intra-abdominal fat. In addition, the smaller the child, the more difficult the localization.

The parenchyma of the testis has a relatively low attenuation and is surrounded by a dense tunica albuginea. The spermatic cord has soft-tissue density and in obese patients, may contain fat. Wolverson *et al.*[32] were able to localize successfully 12 of 15 testes by CT: in two patients the testes were intra-abdominal. One small ultra-abdominal testis was missed on CT but found on surgical exploration. Rajfer *et al.*[34] correctly localized seven impalpable testes, three of which were inside the internal ring in patients aged 10–38 years. In another study of older patients (age range 9–38 years) Lee *et al.*[35] located 7 intra-abdominal or intracanalicular testes.

Not all reports have found CT useful. For example, Green[36] examined 36 testes by CT but could not find them in 16 (44% false-negative rate). There were no false-positive results. In one patient, the CT scan correctly identified an intra-abdominal testis. The effect of age on reliability is yet to be established: to have a major role in the investigation of the impalpable testis, the CT scan must be shown to be effective in accurately identifying the position of a testis at 1 year of age, the age of orchidopexy.

The usefulness of CT scan for identifying intracanalicular testes is offset by the fact that these testes will be readily identified during surgical exploration. As their treatment involves orchidopexy anyway, there is no advantage in performing a CT scan pre-operatively.

6.6.5 Magnetic resonance imaging (MRI)

MRI is a non-invasive, non-ionizing method of locating undescended testes, capable of obtaining multiplanar images. It has been shown to identify clearly bilateral intra-abdominal testes in an adult.[37]

The potential additional benefit of localization of an impalpable testis with MRI is that it may provide information on tissue characteristics. Fritzsche *et al.*[27] found that with prolongation of TR and TE (T2-weighted) sequences, some of the undescended testes were of lower signal intensity than the controlateral descended testis. The significance of these observations is yet to be determined.

The disadvantages to MRI include:

(1) The long scanning time, which is sometimes poorly tolerated by children.
(2) The need for sedation to obtain an optimal study in children under 5 years of age.
(3) The expense, which is significantly higher than that of either ultrasound or CT.
(4) The lack of gastrointestinal contrast media, which makes detection of the intra-abdominal undescended testis difficult.[27]

Despite this, the extra-abdominal testes can apparently be demonstrated in both the coronal and transaxial planes with reasonable reliability, although no large series are currently available. The role of MR imaging may be enhanced by refinements in clinical MR spectroscopy.[38]

6.6.6 Spermatic venography

These techniques are invasive and risk damage to vessels and the testis.[39,40] Venography involves selective catheterization of the testicular vein (gonadal or spermatic vein). It is a relatively invasive and time-consuming technique which has not been adopted widely, although it is probably a fairly reliable tool, if successfully achieved. Selective testicular venography (selective catheterization of the testicular vein) requires technical expertise, a sedative or general anaesthetic for the young child, radiation exposure and a potential risk of morbidity. The key to interpretation is the presence of a pampiniform plexus which almost always indicates a testis is present. A blind-ending testicular vein suggests an absent testis,[41] but occasionally a testicular artery or vas deferens may be present without a normal testicular (gonadal) vein. Incomplete opacification of the testicular vein because of a competent valve or any other technical problem cannot be considered predictive of the presence or absence of a testis.

Green[36] employed spermatic venography in 16 patients (19 testes) in which CT failed to localize the testis. In 32% the procedure could not be accomplished for technical reasons, e.g. inability to cannulate the spermatic vein, and most of these were young children (mean age 4.6 years). Subsequent surgical exploration identified 18 testes, mostly just inside the internal ring.

Selective gonadal venography employs a modified Seldinger technique in which the catheter is introduced into the femoral vein. For the left testicular vein, the catheter is introduced via the left renal vein (requiring two curves), a difficult technique which often requires modification of the shape of the catheter. The right vein is even more difficult to enter because of its location of the antero-lateral wall of the inferior vena cava.

6.6.7 Arteriography

Arteriography has been successful in locating an impalpable testis in adults[42,43] but its use has not been reported in children.[41] Arteriography has a significant morbidity, and causes more discomfort than venography and will probably never be used widely.

6.6.8 Laparoscopy

Rationale

Laparoscopy is based on the assumption that since the vas deferens and epididymis are rarely separated completely from the testis, visualisation of the vas will lead to the testis if it is present.[44]

Proponents of the technique advocate that it is an adjunctive procedure at the time of inguinal-abdominal exploration in boys with an impalpable testis. The age it is performed is the same as that advised for orchidopexy, i.e. currently 1–2 years.

Indications

Routine laparoscopy for impalpable testes allows the surgeon to plan the surgical approach and avoid unnecessary laparotomy.[45] It is perhaps surprising, therefore, as Elder[45] has observed, that the technique is not mentioned in several major textbooks on laparoscopy.[46–48] Naslund *et al.*[49] found that preoperative treatment with hCG made many impalpable testes palpable, obviating the need in these for laparoscopy (and also resulting in a high apparent incidence of 'vanishing testis').

A second indication is in the older child who has undergone previous (but deemed inadequate) inguinal exploration, where either no testis was identified, or where only a vas with no testicular vessels was seen.[45] For example, in one series of 13 patients who had undergone a previous negative inguinal exploration for an impalpable testis, five had an intra-abdominal testis.[50] Duckett[25] has highlighted the problem of previous retroperitoneal exploration through the inguinal canal, where the peritoneum was not opened – in these the intra-abdominal exploration must be considered inadequate, and laparoscopy may be useful.

Laparoscopy may also be indicated in a teenager or adult with an impalpable testis who had not undergone previous exploration.[45]

A baby or child with bilateral impalpable testes, in whom an hCG stimulation test is negative, presents a dilemma, particularly if the penis is respectable in size and responds well to testosterone.[25] Some clinicians would perform laparoscopy in this situation to confirm 'a vanishing testis syndrome',[25] rather than abdominal exploration.

Contraindications

Contraindications to laparoscopy for impalpable testes are summarized as follows:

(1) Absolute:
  (a) Prune-belly syndrome (testes are intra-abdominal).
  (b) Bleeding diathesis.
  (c) Previous abdominal surgery (adhesions).
(2) Relative:
  (a) Obesity.
  (b) Umbilical hernia (can use more inferior incision).

Technique of laparoscopy

The bladder is emptied. With the child supine and under general anaesthesia, the abdomen is insufflated with carbon dioxide using a Verres needle. The amount depends on the size of the child (between 0.05 and 1.5 litre). Over-distension causes ventilatory difficulty. If the pressure is greater than 20 mm Hg, the needle is in an incorrect position. A trochar is inserted just below the umbilicus through which a Storz paediatric laparoscope is inserted. The abdomen and each paracolic gutter is visualized in turn by tilting the child away from the side to be examined and in 15–20° Trendelenburg. A normal vas running from the pelvis to the internal ring converges with the gonadal vessels at the internal inguinal ring; if this is seen groin exploration is undertaken, as the testis is located in the inguinal canal. If there is no vas visible the paracolic gutters are examined to look for a testis. If the vas and vessels end abruptly, it is suggestive of antenatal or early postnatal torsion, the so called intra-abdominal vanishing testis.

Cperative findings

A number of observations can be made at laparoscopy (Table 6.1). In the

Table 6.1 The impalpable testis: laparoscopic findings

Series	Number of impalable gonads	Location of gonad		
		Intra-abdominal	Canalicular	Absent
Scott[59]	24	10	–	12
Lowe *et al.*[55]	36	14	12	10
Boddy *et al.*[50]	55	19	7	29
Manson *et al.*[56]	17	5	11	1
Weiss and Seashore[57]	33	5	7	21
Guiney *et al.*[51]	103	53	11	39
Bloom *et al.*[58]	28	11	7	10

large study by Guiney *et al.*[51] it was found that 39% of impalpable testes were absent on laparoscopy, and the majority of the remainder (53 out of 64) were visible within the abdomen.

The primary objective is to see the internal ring.[51] When the testis has descended beyond the internal ring, the retroperitoneal leash of testicular vessels is joined by the whitish vas deferens as a 'V' at this ring and has a characteristic appearance. When the testis is impalpable, the commonest finding is that of a testis that is readily seen lying within a centimeter or two of the internal ring. If the intra-abdominal testis is not immediately apparent it can be traced by following the testicular vessels; and if the vessels appear much smaller than normal, and their course takes them into the internal canal, it is likely that there is no testis present. If the vessels and blind-ending vas deferens lie contiguously – the so-called 'vanishing testis' – then at some time in embryological development, a testis was probably present.[52]

Very occasionally, there may be no evidence of a vas or vessels within the accessible peritoneal cavity. This suggests true congenital absence of the testis and extensive dissection up to the lower pole of the kidney will be unrewarding.[51]

Complications

The complications of laparoscopy may be summarized as follows:

(1) Incorrect placement of needle or trochar:
  - (a) Extraperitoneal insufflation.
  - (b) Omental emphysema.
  - (c) Perforation of bladder or bowel.
  - (d) Injury to pelvic veins or arteries.

(2) Excessive insufflation:
  - (a) Ventilatory difficulty.
  - (b) Mediastinal emphysema.

(3) Failure to visualize vas, testicular vessels or gonad.
(4) Abdominal pain following laparoscopy.
(5) Bleeding from abdominal wall.
(6) Gas embolism.

The most common complication of laparoscopy is extraperitoneal insufflation of air and subcutaneous emphysema, due to failure of the Verres needle to enter the peritoneal cavity.[53] A related problem is omental emphysema, which should be considered when the insufflation pressure is high.[45] The three main causes of complications are (1) poor placement of the Verres needle; (2) improper ventilation of the patient resulting in hypercarbia and hypoxia; and (3) excessive intra-abdominal pressure (greater than 20 mm Hg).[53] The complication rate is lowest when laparoscopy is performed by surgeons who perform more than 60 procedures per year.[54]

6.6.9 Surgical exploration

In many centres, including our own, primary exploration for an impalpable testis is performed without prior radiological or laparoscopic investigation. If the infant or child has bilateral impalpable testes, an hCG stimulation test will have been performed. In unilateral cryptorchidism, the operation is commenced in the knowledge that the testis will be either in the abdomen, in the inguinal canal or absent. The technique of surgical exploration is described in Chapter 7.

6.7 Conclusion

In many centres, there is a trend towards radiological investigation of patients with both unilateral and bilateral impalpable testes. Unfortunately, for the testis for which accurate localization would be useful, i.e. the intra-abdominal testis, the techniques are either ineffective and unreliable, or expensive, or both. Reports describing the use of these techniques refer to a significant number of patients in whom the testes are distal to the inguinal canal, suggesting that they may have, in fact, been palpable to an experienced clinician.

The first step, therefore, in the management of a patient in whom a testis is not palpable should be referral to a specialist who is skilled in examining the inguinal region in a boy: this is usually a paediatric surgeon.[31] Many previously 'impalpable' testes then become 'palpable', and no further pre-operative investigation is required.

Laparoscopy is another investigation which is being used. Although it is invasive, requires general anaesthesia and is time consuming, it has a high degree of reliability and accuracy, and can be performed under the same anaesthetic as the subsequent orchidopexy (when indicated).

The mainstay of localization remains surgical exploration: intracanalicular testes are identified readily and the intra-abdominal testis can be localized by opening the peritoneum at the internal inguinal ring or by following the retroperitoneal course of the vas deferens. The surgeon should be aware of the rare situation of complete separation of the testis and vas deferens, and absence of the testis.

References

1. Wyllie GG. The diagnosis of the undescended testis. *Med J Aust* 1978; **i:** 639–41.
2. Scorer CG. The incidence of incomplete descent of the testicle at birth. *Arch Dis Child* 1956; **31:** 330–32.
3. Scorer CG. Descent of the testis. *Arch Dis Child* 1964; **39:** 605.
4. John Radcliffe Hospital Study Group. Clinical diagnosis of cryptorchidism. *Arch Dis Child* 1988; **63:** 587–91.
5. Scorer CG, Farrington GH. *Congenital Deformities of the Testis and Epididymis.* New York: Appleton-Century-Crofts, 1971: p. 184.
6. Johansen TEB, Larmo A. Ultrasound in the evaluation of retractile and truly undescended testes. *Scand J Urol Nephrol* 1988; **22:** 245–50.
7. Fenton E, Woodward AA, Hudson IL, Marschner I. The ascending testis. *Pediatr Surg Int* 1990; **4:** 6–9
8. Atwell JD. Ascent of the testis: fact or fiction? *Br J Urol* 1985; **57:** 474–7.
9. Kaplan GW. Editorial comment. *J Urol* 1985; **143:** 368.
10. Karpe B. Prognosis of hormonal treatment of undescended testis related to testicular position at birth. *Pediatr Surg Int* 1991; **6:** 221–2.
11. Coplan MM, Woods FM, Melvin PD. The perineal testis. *S Med J* 1957; **50:** 1338–46.
12. Jones AE, Lieberthal F. Perineal testicle. *J Urol* 1938; **40:** 658.
13. Wills I. Perineal ectopia. *S Clin N Am* 1934; **14:** 1547.
14. Rea CE. The perineal testis. *Ann Surg* 1938; **108:** 1083.
15. Waffenburgh CA, Rape MG, Beare JB. Perineal testicle. *J Urol.* 1949; **62:** 858.
16. Stirk DI. Strangulated inguinofemoral hernia with descent of the testis through the femoral canal. *Br J Surg* 1955; **43:** 331–2.
17. McEwan JAC. Abnormal descent of the testicle. *Lancet* 1920; **1:** 655–6.
18. Faunteroy AM. Development of an inguinal hernia through the femoral ring following descent of the testicle by the same route. *Ann Surg* 1920; **72:** 675.
19. Beasley SW, Auldist AW. Crossed testicular ectopia in association with double incomplete testicular descent. *Aust NZ J Surg* 1985; **55:** 301–3.
20. Von der Leyden UE. Eine seltene angeborene Fahllagerung des Hodens. *Chirung* 1963: **34:** 521.
21. Heyns CF. Exstrophy of the testis. *J Urol* 1990; **144:** 724–5.
22. Williams DW. Anomaly of scrotum and testes: simple plastic repair. *J Urol* 1963; **89:** 860–3.
23. Adair E, Lewis E. Ectopic scrotum and diphallia: Report of a case. *J Urol* 1960; **84:** 115–7.
24. Campbell HE. Incidence of malignant growth of the undescended testicle. A critical statistical study. *Arch Surg* 1942; **44:** 353–69.
25. Duckett JW. Laparoscopy for cryptorchidism. In: Laparoscopy: its role in the management of nonpalpable testis. *Dial Pediatr Urol* 1988; **11:** 6–7.

26. Madrazo BL, Klugo RC, Parks JA, Diloreto R. Ultrasonographic demonstration of undescended testes. *Ultrasound* 1979; **133:** 181–3.
27. Fritzsche PJ, Hricak H, Kogan BA, Winkler ML, Tanagho EA. Undescended testis: value of MR Imaging. *Radiology* 1987; **164:** 169–73.
28. Hederstrom E, Forsberg L, Kullendorff CM. Ultrasonography of the undescended testis. *Acta Rad Diag* 1985; **26:** 453–6.
29. Weiss RM, Carter AR, Rosenfield AT. High resolution real-time ultrasonagraphy in the localization of the undescended testis. *J Urol* 1986; **135:** 936–8.
30. Graif M, Czerniak A, Avigad I, Strauss S, Wolfstein I. High-resolution sonography of the undescended testis in childhood: an analysis of 45 cases. *Isr J Med Sci* 1990; **26:** 382–5.
31. Barker A, Ahmed S, Freeman JK. Unnecessary investigations for impalpable testes. *Med J Aust* 1987; **147:** 211.
32. Wolverson MK, Jagannadharo, Sundaram B, Riaz MA, Nalesnik WJ, Houttuin E. CT in localization of impalpable cryptorchid testes. *Am J Radiol* 1980; **134:** 725–9.
33. Lee JKT, Glazer HS. Computed tomography in the localization of the non palpable testis. *Urol Clin N Am* 1982; **9:** 397–404.
34. Rajfer J, Tauber A, Zinner N, Naftulin E, Worthen N. The use of computerized scanning to localize the impalpable testis. *J Urol* 1983; **129:** 972–4.
35. Lee JAT, McClonnan BL, Stanley RJ, Sagel SS. Utility of computed tomography in the localization of the undescended testes. *Radiology* 1980; **135:** 121–5.
36. Green CL. Computerized axial tomography vs. spermatic venography in localization of cryptorchid testes. *Urology* 1985; **XXVI:** 513–7.
37. Troughton AH, Waring J, Longstaff A, Goddard PR. The role of magnetic resonance imaging in the investigation of undescended testes. *Clin Radiol* 1990; **41:** 178–81.
38. Bretan PN, Vigneron DB, Hricak H, *et al.* Assessment of testicular metabolic integrity with P-31 MR spectroscopy. *Radiology* 1987; **162:** 867–71.
39. Kahademi M, Seebode JJ, Falla A. Selective spermatic arteriography for localization of an impalpable undescended testis. *Radiology* 1980; **136:** 627–4.
40. Domellof L, Hjalmas K, Nordmark L, Nyberg G. Angiography of the testicular artery as a diagnostic aid in boys with nonpalpable testis. *J Pediatr Surg* 1978; **13:** 534–6.
41. Weiss RM, Glickman MG. Venography of the undescended testis. *Urol Clin N Am* 1982; **9:** 387–95.
42. Ben-Menachem V, de Bevardinis MC, Salinas R. Localization of intra-abdominal testes by selective testicular arteriography: a case report. *J Urol* 1974; **112:** 493.
43. Nordmark L, Bjersing L, Domellof L, Hjalmas K, Nyberg G. Angiography of the testicular artery. II. Cryptorchidism and testicular agenisis. *Acta Radiol Diagn* 1977; **18:** 167.
44. Doig CM. Use of laparoscopy in children with impalpable testes. *Int J Androl* 1980; **12:** 420–2.
45. Elder JS. Laparoscopy and Fowler–Stephens orchiopexy in the management of the impalpable testis. *Urol Clin N Am* 1989; **16:** 399–411.
46. Borten M. *Laparoscopic Complications: Prevention and Management*. Toronto: B C Decker, 1986.
47. Salah JW. *Laparoscopy*. Philadelphia: W B Saunders, 1988.
48. Hulka JF. *Textbook of Laparoscopy*. Orlando, FL: Grune & Stratton, 1985.
49. Naslund MJ, *et al.* Laparoscopy; its selected use in patients with unilateral

nonpalpable testis after human chorionic gonadotropin stimulation. *J Urol* 1989; **142:** 108–10.
50. Boddy SAM, Corkery JJ, Gornall R. The place of laparoscopy in the management of the impalpable testis. *Br J Surg* 1985; **72:** 918–9.
51. Guiney EJ, *et al.* Laparoscopy and the management of the impalpable testis. *Br J Urol* 1989; **63:** 313–6.
52. Abeyaratine M, Aherne W, Scott J. The vanishing testis. *Lancet* 1969; **ii:** 882–4.
53. de Cherney A. Complications in laparoscopy. In: Laparoscopy: its role in the management of nonpalpable testis. *Dial Pediatr Urol* 1988; **11:** 7–8.
54. Phillips JM, Keith D, Keith L, *et al.* Survey of gynaecological laparoscopy for 1974. *J Reprod Med* 1975; **15:** 45.
55. Lowe DH, Brock WA, Kaplan GW. Laparoscopy for localization of nonpalpable testes. *J Urol* 1984; **131:** 728–9.
56. Manson AL, Terhume D, Jordan G, Auman JR, Peterson N, MacDonald G. Preoperative laparoscopic localization of the nonpalpable testis. *J Urol* 1985; **134:** 919–20.
57. Weiss RM, Seashore JH. Laparoscopy in the management of the nonpalpable testis. *J Urol* 1987; **138:** 382–4.
58. Bloom DA, Ayers JTW, McGuire EJ. The role of laparotomy in management of nonpalpable testes. *J d'Urol* 1988; **94:** 465.
59. Scott JES. Laparoscopy as an aid in the diagnosis and management of the impalpable testis. *J Pediatr Surg* 1982; **17:** 14–16.

7

Operative treatment

7.1 Planning surgery

Surgery is currently the only effective and reliable way of bringing the undescended testis into the scrotum; this chapter describes in detail the surgical procedures that can be employed. Orchidopexy is usually a straightforward procedure, but occasionally the short length of spermatic cord available, or the flimsy inverting hernial sac (particularly with the intracanalicular testis) may create operative difficulty. On other occasions, the presence of testicular–epididymal fusion abnormalities, the 'vanishing testis', polyorchidism, absent vas, splenogonadal fusion or ectopic (adrenal or renal) tissue, may cause confusion. The recognition and management of these unusual and difficult situations is discussed.

Meticulous attention to operative technique with careful separation of the processus vaginalis or hernial sac, and exact dissection of the cord to increase its length, contribute to the good results now expected after orchidopexy. Orchidopexy is best performed by trained paediatric surgeons who are familiar with handling infantile tissue, and who feel comfortable operating with loupe glasses. The 'occasional orchidopexy' is not an operation which adult general surgeons should be encouraged to perform, unless there are no paediatric surgical facilities available.

7.1.1 Age at orchidopexy

When paediatric surgery first became a specialty, orchidopexies were performed in the prepubertal child. Since then, there has been a stepwise fall in the age at which orchidopexy has been advocated (Figure 7.1),

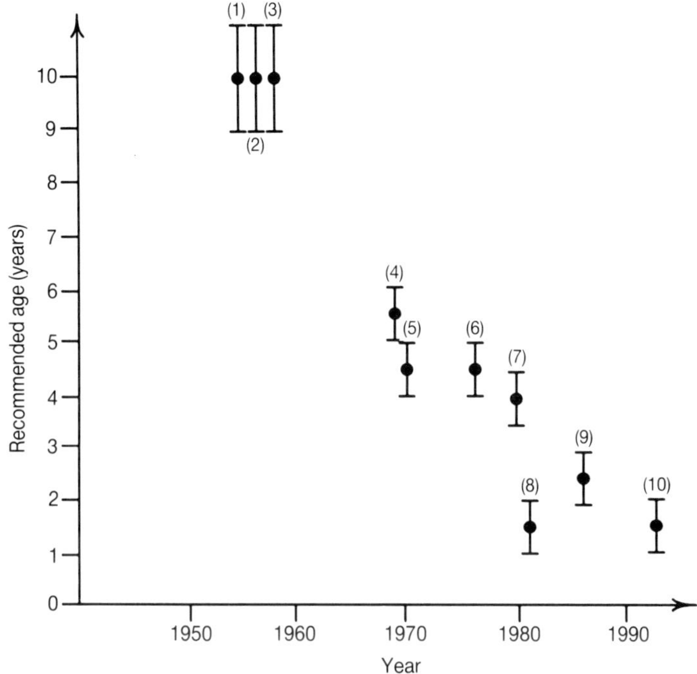

Figure 7.1 The age at which orchidopexy has been advocated since the 1950s. (1) Gross and Jewett[54]; (2) Swenson[55]; (3) Potts[56]; (4) Snyder and Greaney[57]; (5) Jones[58]; (6) Jones[59]; (7) Campbell[60]; (8) Fonkalsrud and Mengel[61]; (9) Jones and Woodward[62]; (10) Hutson *et al.*[63]

mainly as a result of the histological evidence of testicular damage which occurs in the untreated undescended testis after infancy.[1] The age at which orchidopexy is best performed is now believed to be about 12 months, and certainly before 3 years, prior to morphological damage to the undescended testis. The effect of late orchidopexy on fertility has been discussed in Chapter 5. At present it is not known whether this policy of early surgery will improve the current prognosis. Insufficient time has elapsed since implementation of the suggestion that surgery be done in infancy, for the long-term outcome on fertility and malignancy to be known (Chapter 9).

If a clinically evident hernia appears in an infant who has an ipsilateral undescended testis, an orchidopexy should be performed at the same time as the herniotomy, irrespective of the age of the infant. Failure to do so would make subsequent orchidopexy extremely difficult, owing to fibrous adhesions in the region of the internal ring.

Good paediatric surgical technique, facilitated by the use of loupe (magnifying) glasses, means that orchidopexy can be performed with great accuracy and safety in infants and in small children. Despite this, however, concurrent orchidopexy in an infant who requires a herniotomy for a symptomatic hernia, remains a demanding operation. There is some, as yet only preliminary, evidence to suggest that the testes may be best brought down earlier than 12 months: müllerian inhibiting substance levels normally peak between 4 and 12 months in infants with cryptorchidism; these levels appear to be inhibited (Figure 5.5, page 81).[2] These results suggest early physiological derangement in the undescended testis prior to the morphological abnormality seen at 12–24 months.

Repeated careful examination of children with markedly retractile testes may identify the occasional child demonstrating 'ascent' of the testis – this testis should be brought down at the time it is first recognized to have become 'cryptorchid'.

Likewise, the child who first presents during later childhood will have his orchidopexy performed shortly after the age of presentation. Even though recent teaching has advocated orchidopexy well before the age of 3 years, referral of cryptorchid patients occurs throughout childhood (se Figure 4.6, page 58). This highlights both the importance of the ongoing education of the primary medical practitioner (and of the community at large), and the possibility that many 'undescended' testes may be acquired.

7.1.2 The day surgical procedure

Orchidopexy is now performed as a day surgical procedure. The child is admitted to the day surgical ward an hour or so before surgery, where he is re-examined and seen by the anaesthetist. In most centres, the parents remain with the child until he is asleep, and are again present once he leaves the operating or procedure room. The child does not require a bed until the anaesthetic is commenced, and is usually 'held' in a room specially designed for children, with TV or video facilities and a range of appropriate toys and play activities. This reduces pre-operative anxiety and obviates the need for pre-medication.

The child is allowed to leave the day surgical facility once he is fully awake from the anaesthetic. It is not necessary to wait until he has passed urine or been fed. Where local or regional anaesthetic agents have been used, it is preferable to have the boy home before their effect has worn off. The parents – and the child, if old enough – should be informed of the likely intensity and duration of post-operative discomfort. Use of subcuticular absorbable sutures means that the child does not have to cope with the anxiety and trauma of suture removal. Waterproof dressings (e.g. Tegaderm and Opsite) allow normal bathing and water activities in the early post-operative period and avoid the need for wound care. The ultimate cosmetic result for an incision made in the lap crease is excellent.

7.1.3 Anaesthesia

The type of anaesthetic offered children undergoing orchidopexy reflects the day surgical nature of the procedure. The aim of the anaesthesia is not only to have the child totally unaware of the operation taking place, but also to have him wake up quickly and fully, to be in little discomfort, so that he may go home promptly and with minimal psychological and physical trauma.

Pre-medication
In most boys, no pre-medication is required. The provision of enlightened 'child-friendly' day surgical facilities, and the acceptance of parents being with the child right up to and including induction of anaesthesia, remove most of the anxiety and agitation which previously necessitated the use of pre-medication agents.

If a 'pre-med' is to be given, oral preparations (e.g. chloral hydrate) are preferable to intramuscular injections, because children are fearful of needles.

Instead of a pre-med, it is better to apply EMLA cream (Astra Pharmaceuticals) to the back of the hand so that when the intravenous inducing agent is to be given, the child will experience no pain. Indeed, if distracted to look the other way, he will usually be unaware that intravenous access has been obtained.

Use of regional or local anaesthesia
An ilio-inguinal nerve block or local anaesthetic injected into the wound edges provide satisfactory pain relief for the first few hours postoperatively.

7.2 The standard orchidopexy

The standard orchidopexy for a palpable testis involves an inguinal incision, full exposure of the inguinal canal, separation of the processus vaginalis or hernial sac, mobilization of the cord structures and scrotal fixation of the testis in a subdartos pouch. Trans-scrotal orchidopexy[3] has not gained widespread acceptance.

7.2.1 Approach to inguinal canal

The inguinal canal is approached through a transverse lap crease incision (Figure 7.2) and the wound deepened to Scarpa's fascia. Diathermy dissection achieves this with minimal blood loss (Figure 7.3). In an infant or small child Scarpa's fascia is a relatively well formed and substantial pale membrane, which can be distinguished from the external oblique

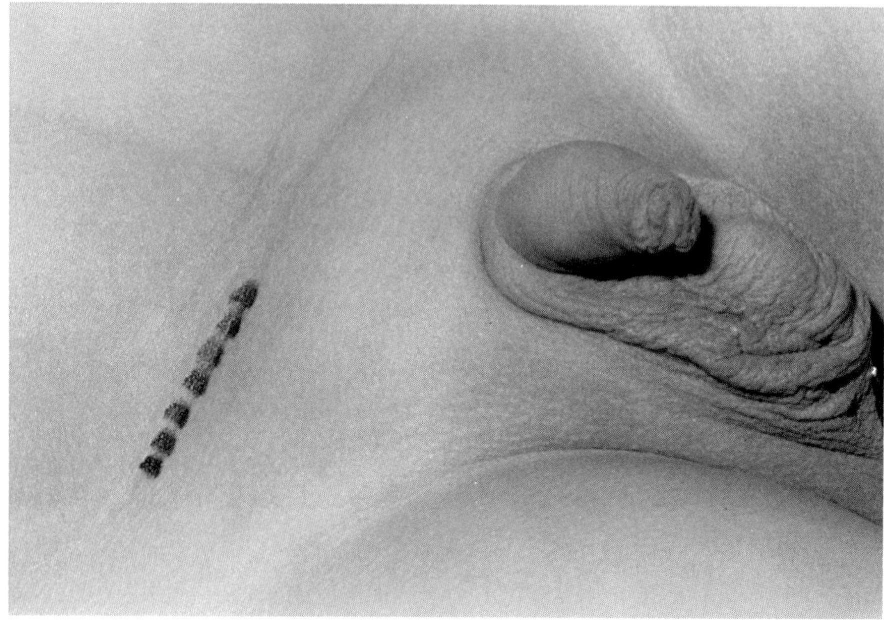

Figure 7.2 The incision for orchidopexy is made through the transverse lap skin crease.

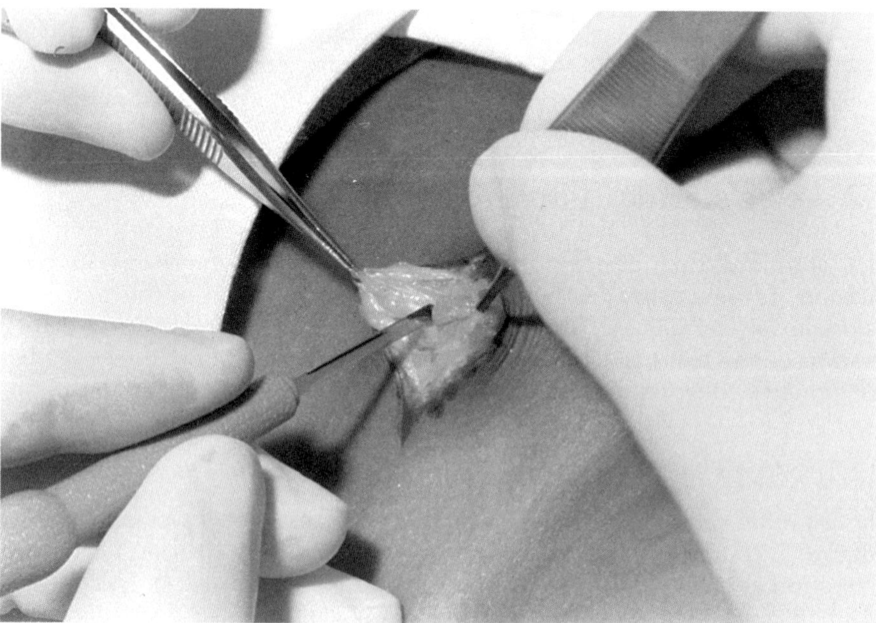

Figure 7.3 The subcutaneous tissue and Scarpa's fascia can be divided by diathermy dissection, causing minimal blood loss.

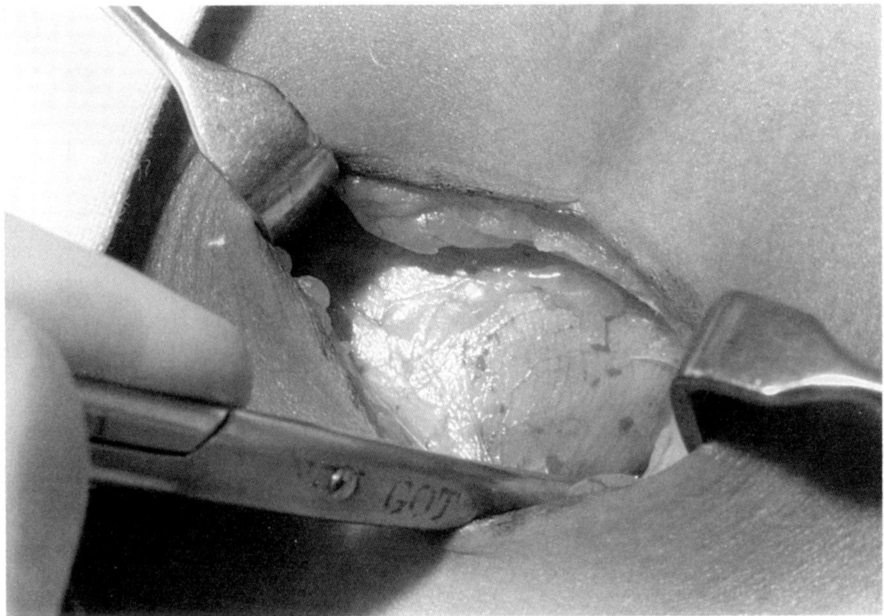

Figure 7.4 The anterior surface of the external oblique aponeurosis is exposed inferiorly as far as the inguinal ligament by using a sweeping movement with closed scissors.

aponeurosis by its absence of oblique fibres. Once Scarpa's fascia has been incised the wound can be developed and exposed using square-ended retractors: this dissection is continued as far as the external oblique aponeurosis itself. A sweeping motion parallel to the line of the external oblique with scissors separates the fascial and subcutaneous layers form the aponeurosis as far as the inguinal ligament inferiorly (Figure 7.4).

When this sweeping movement is continued medially the bifurcation of the fibres of the external oblique aponeurosis at the external inguinal ring, and the bulge of the spermatic cord become apparent. The inguinal canal can be exposed by either incising the external oblique aponeurosis laterally in line with the external ring and cutting along the fibres towards the ring (Figure 7.5) or by cutting laterally along the fibres from the external ring.

7.2.2 Identification of testis

The approximate position of the testis will usually be known prior to surgery. In the most common situation where the testis is in the region of the external inguinal ring and overlying the pubic bone, it will be observed first during the approach to the inguinal canal. Within its processus vaginalis that extends from the external ring, it is often situated

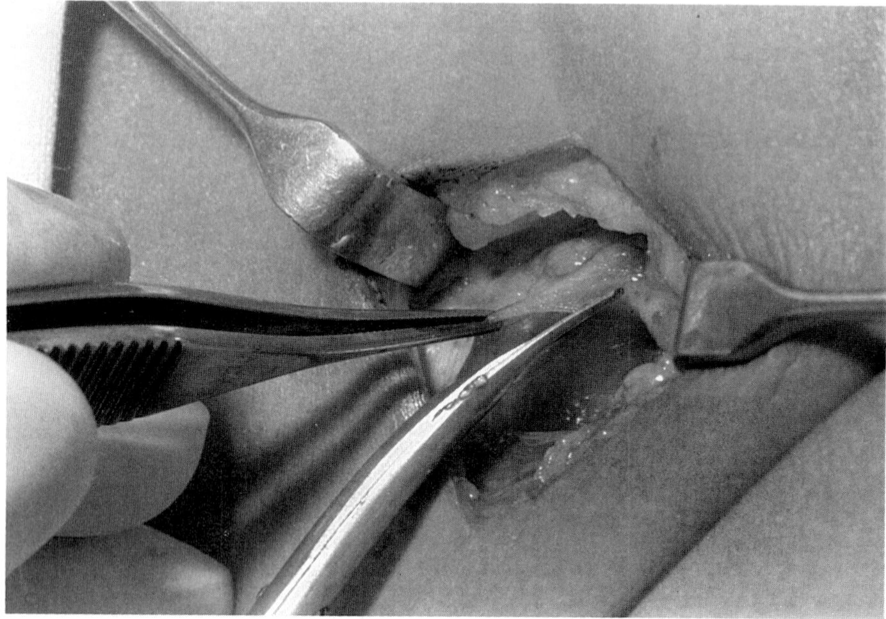

Figure 7.5 Exposure of the inguinal canal is achieved by incising the fibres of the external oblique aponeurosis to open the external inguinal ring.

immediately superficial to the external oblique aponeurosis. Care should be taken to avoid its damage during opening of the inguinal canal.

Where its position is not immediately obvious, it can be traced by following the spermatic cord as it continues through the external inguinal ring. Where the testis has been impalpable clinically, it may not be located until the inguinal canal is opened where it will be found either within the inguinal canal or within the abdomen (see later section).

7.2.3 Separation of gubernaculum

A gubernaculum can be found at operation in all patients with undescended testes,[4] and is attached to a site other than the lower scrotum in most. In undescended testes the gubernaculum appears to have an abnormal attachment, usually lateral to or above the neck of the scrotum (Figure 7.6). This can be demonstrated when the testis is lifted out of the wound to place tension on the gubernaculum which then causes the skin adjacent to its attachment to become dimpled.

The testis should be separated from the gubernaculum by teasing the gubernaculum off the tunica vaginalis with broad blunt forceps. If performed at the right level close to the tunical attachment, this procedure is bloodless. This allows the testis to be lifted out of the wound and enables

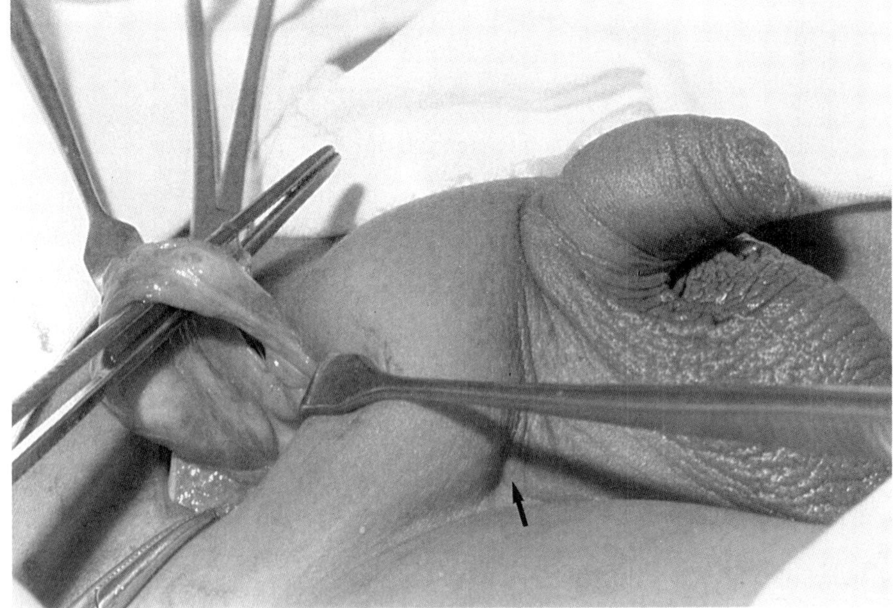

Figure 7.6 The abnormal attachment of the gubernaculum in cryptorchidism, here causing dimpling above and lateral to the neck of the scrotum (arrow). The forceps are lifting the testis and cord structures upwards out of the wound. The gubernaculum is then separated from the testis.

the cremaster muscle to be stripped off the spermatic cord (Figure 7.7). Sometimes it contains small vessels which require diathermy.

7.2.4 The hernial sac

In the great majority of boys with cryptorchidism there is a widely patent processus vaginalis.[5,6] The width of the processus vaginalis is often of such size that it is interpreted as being a hernial sac,[4] even though in the vast majority there will not have been a symptomatic hernia. In a study of 68 testes, Jackson *et al.*[4] found a clearly identifiable 'hernial sac' in 35 (51.5%) although at what point a patent processus vaginalis becomes a hernial sac is purely subjective. Scorer documented a 'hernia' in 55%[7] and Heath *et al.*[8] in 21.2%. It should be acknowledged that the incidence of a hernial sac in otherwise normal boys is unknown. By contrast, in our experience, complete absence of an identifiable processus vaginalis is extremely unusual. Nevertheless, the exact relationship to, and significance of, a hernia in cryptorchidism is argued.[9,10]

There is no argument that separation of the hernial sac (patent processus vaginalis) from the vas deferens and testicular vessels increases the effective length of the cord during orchidopexy.

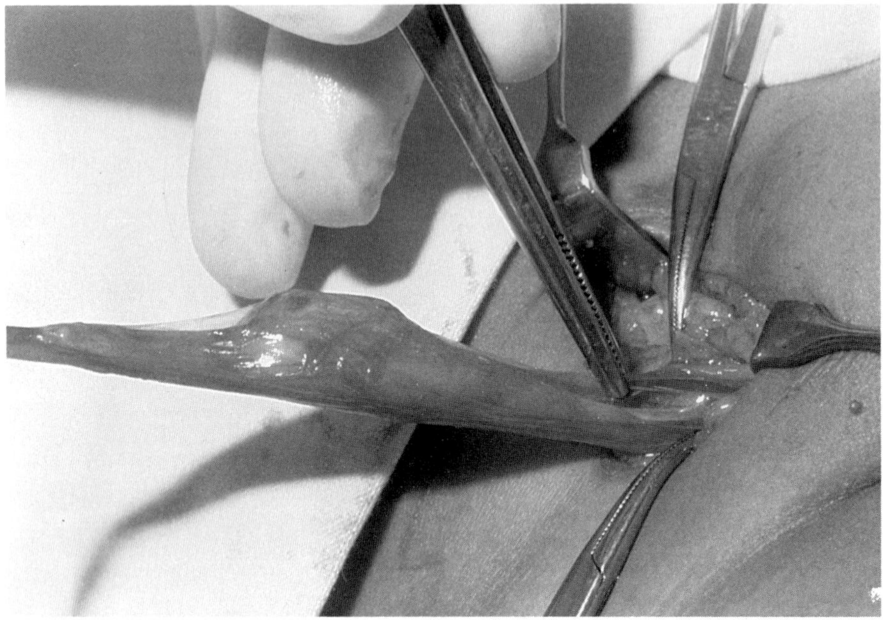

Figure 7.7 The testis and cord are pulled out of the wound with traction, allowing the cremaster muscle fibres to be stripped off the cord.

The method of separation of the sac is the same as that employed during routine herniotomy: the sac is stretched over the index finger while the round-ended non-toothed dissecting forceps gently sweep off the other cord structures, or the sac can be held in forceps while the vessels and vas are isolated *en masse* off the sac. In this way the sac is completely separated from the cord (Figure 7.8).

At no stage are either the vas deferens or vessels held by the forceps; otherwise they may be damaged. The technique of separation is achieved most efficiently if the sac remains intact. Inadvertent opening of the sac should be recognized early to prevent extension of the tear through the internal ring into the peritoneum, where its closure becomes technically more difficult.

The vas deferens has a tendency to remain with the sac; so it must be ensured that it is seen with the vessels before the sac is divided.

Once the structures of the spermatic cord have been separated from the sac, the sac is divided (Figure 7.9). The sac is then dissected proximally well into the internal ring (Figure 7.10). As the processus vaginalis becomes peritoneum, its appearance changes from transparent to white and its base widens into a triangular structure. At this level the vas deferens can be observed to be deviating medially towards the base of the bladder while the testicular vessels continue straight into the

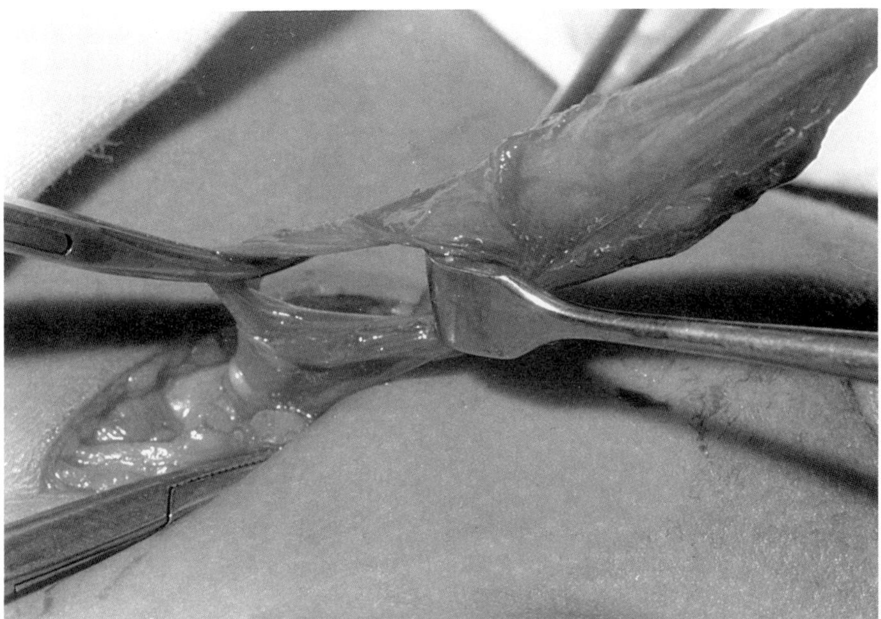

Figure 7.8 The widely patent processus vaginalis (hernial sac) is separated from the remaining cord structures in the same way as in a routine herniotomy.

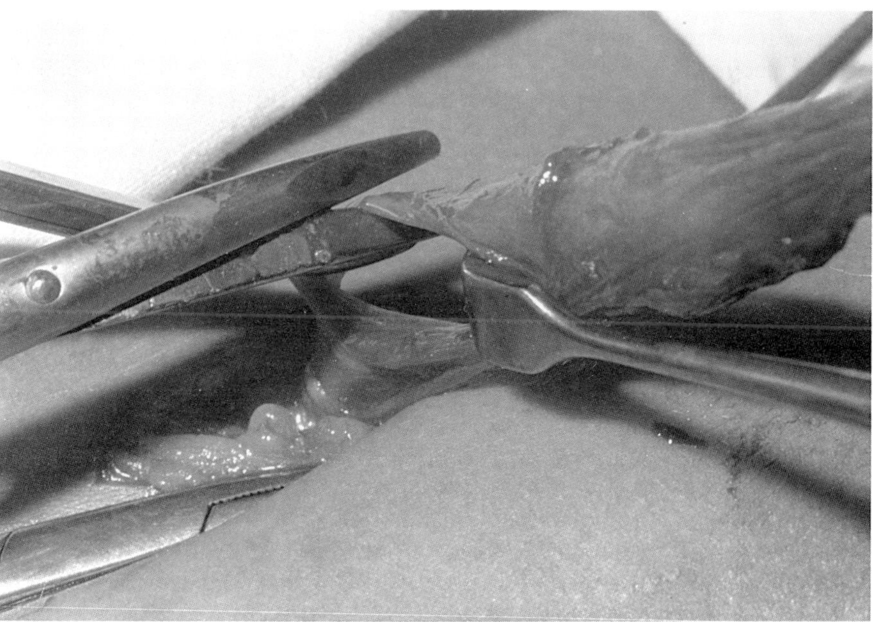

Figure 7.9 Once completely separated from the vas deferens and testicular vessels, the sac is divided with scissors.

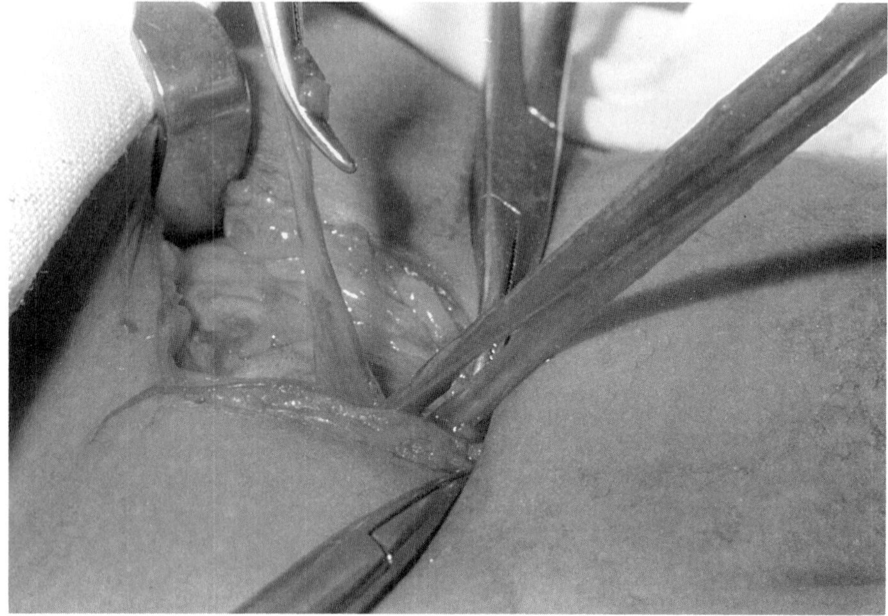

Figure 7.10 Dissection of the sac is then continued to the internal inguinal ring. Note the commencement of the separation of the vas deferens (running medially) and the vessels (running more laterally) at the internal ring.

retroperitoneum in a more lateral position. Extraperitoneal fat is found once dissection reaches above the internal inguinal ring. The hernial sac is transfixed at the internal ring (Figure 7.11).

7.2.5 Freeing the vessels and vas

As the testicular artery tracks downwards in the posterior abdominal wall from its origin on the aorta, it crosses the pelvic inlet and follows a gentle curve around the postero-lateral concavity of the pelvic cavity to reach the internal inguinal ring, just lateral to the inferior epigastric artery. In doing so, it has thin bands of loose and relatively avascular connective tissue which attach it to the wall of the pelvis; these bands can be demonstrated at surgery when traction is placed on the vessels after separation of the processus vaginalis. Their division, by straightening the path taken by the vessels, effectively lengthens the spermatic cord and allows the testis to reach the scrotum (Figure 7.12). They can be divided easily by blunt dissection with non-toothed forceps (by 'teasing' them off the cord) or by sharp dissection with scissors, taking extreme care to avoid damage to the testicular vessels themselves.

Once the manoeuvre is completed, the cord should be fully mobilized with the vas seen curving around the inferior epigastric vessels as it

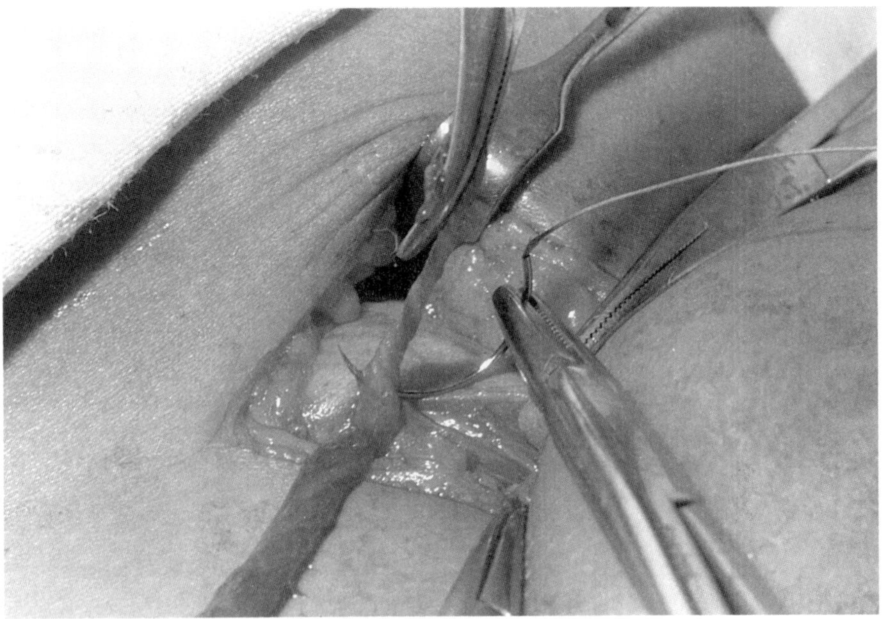

Figure 7.11 The hernial sac is transfixed at the internal ring only after it has been fully separated from the remaining cord structures.

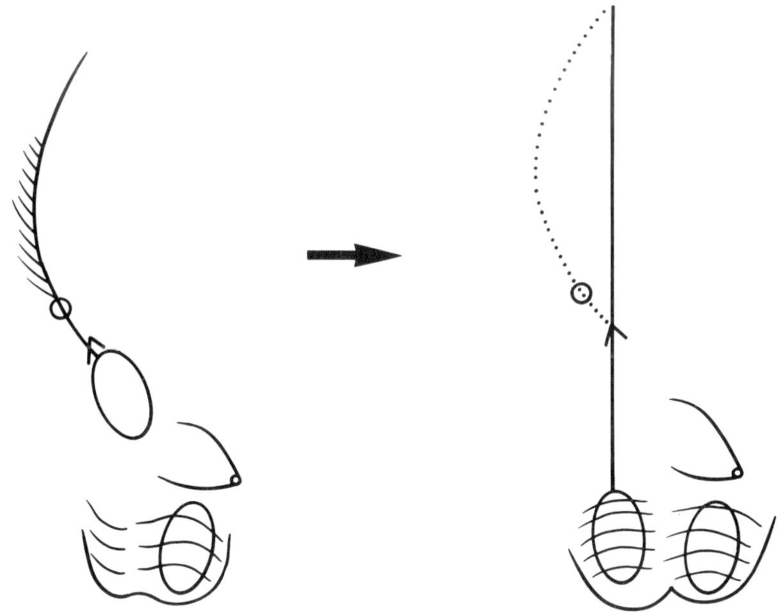

Figure 7.12 Division of lateral avascular attachments of the cord proximal to the internal ring allows the path taken by the spermatic cord to be more direct, effectively lengthening that part of the cord beyond the internal inguinal ring.

runs towards the base of the bladder, and the testicular artery and its accompanying veins free from the lateral pelvic wall, and running straight upwards into the retroperitoneum (Figure 7.13).

As a rule, the vas deferens has sufficient length to reach the scrotum easily.[11]

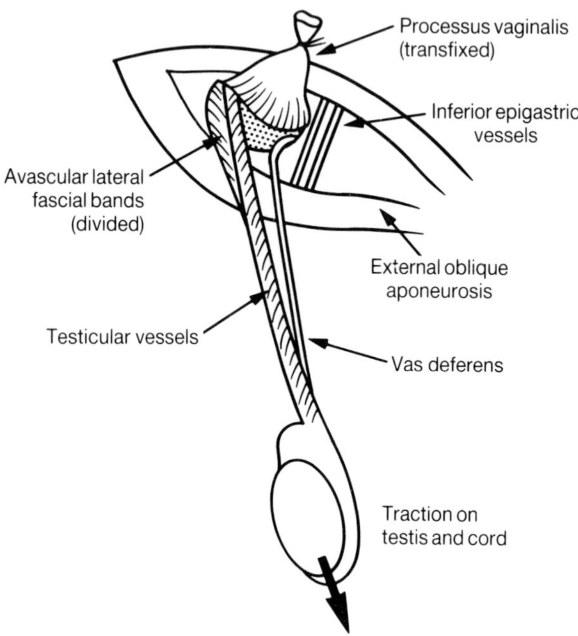

Figure 7.13 The vas deferens bends medially around the inferior epigastric artery at the internal ring, whereas the vessels follow a straighter course through the ring.

7.2.6 Placement of testis in scrotum

After the testis and cord has been adequately mobilized, the testis is placed in the scrotum. This is achieved by first creating a space in the scrotum in which the testis and epididymis can be situated. A midline or transverse scrotal incision is made to gain access to the subdartos space in which the plane is developed by divulsion using scissors or forceps (Figure 7.14). Some authors[11,12] describe a pouch in the scrotum between the skin and dartos. Given the attachment of the dartos muscle in the scrotal skin, and the absence of muscle deep to this plane in which creation of a pouch is possible, it is likely that they are describing what could more correctly be called a subdartos pouch. Bleeding points are controlled by diathermy. The index finger or a mosquito forcep is then introduced from above along the path intended for the testis, to guide another forcep from below, which

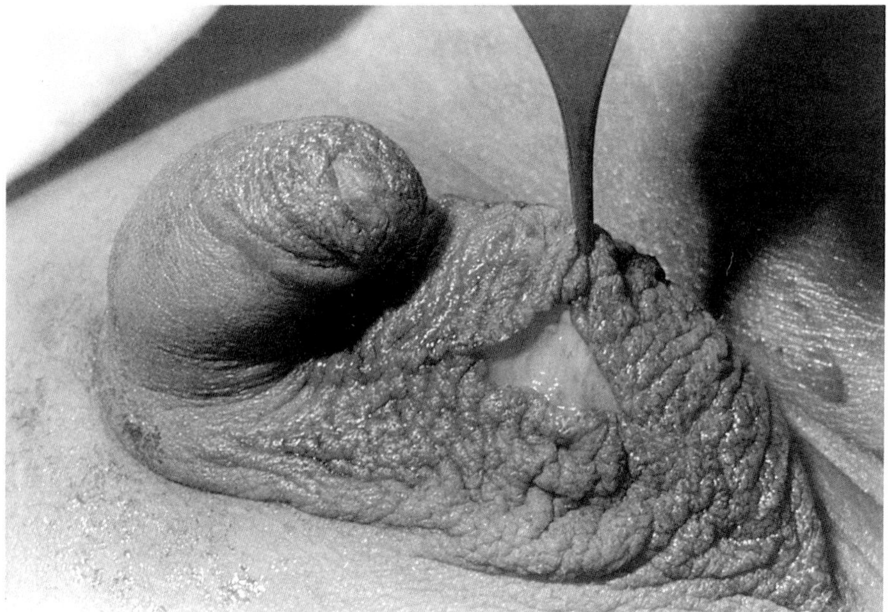

Figure 7.14 Midline scrotal incision and creation of a sub-dartos pouch.

is used to grasp the distal tunical coverings of the testis, which are then drawn gently down the track through the 'button-hole' in the subdartos pouch, into the scrotum (Figure 7.15). The forceps do not hold the testis itself, thus avoiding direct trauma to the gonad.

7.2.7 Fixation of the testis

When the testis is placed into the scrotum, it has to be pulled through the loose fascial layers at the neck of the scrotum. If there is no tension on the cord, this alone will prevent subsequent upwards retraction of the testis. Alternatively, the testis can be anchored to the midline tissue of the scrotum by a 3/0 suture through the tunica albuginea (Figure 7.16), or the fascial tissues of the neck of the scrotum can be closed to prevent retraction of the testis, taking care to avoid constriction of the testicular vessels. A theoretical advantage of direct anchorage of the testis is in reducing the likelihood (albeit rare) of subsequent torsion.[13] The scrotum is closed with 4/0 subcuticular absorbable sutures.

7.2.8 Dressings and after-care

The use of subcuticular absorbable sutures means that no sutures require removal post-operatively (which is in the child's interests) and ensures

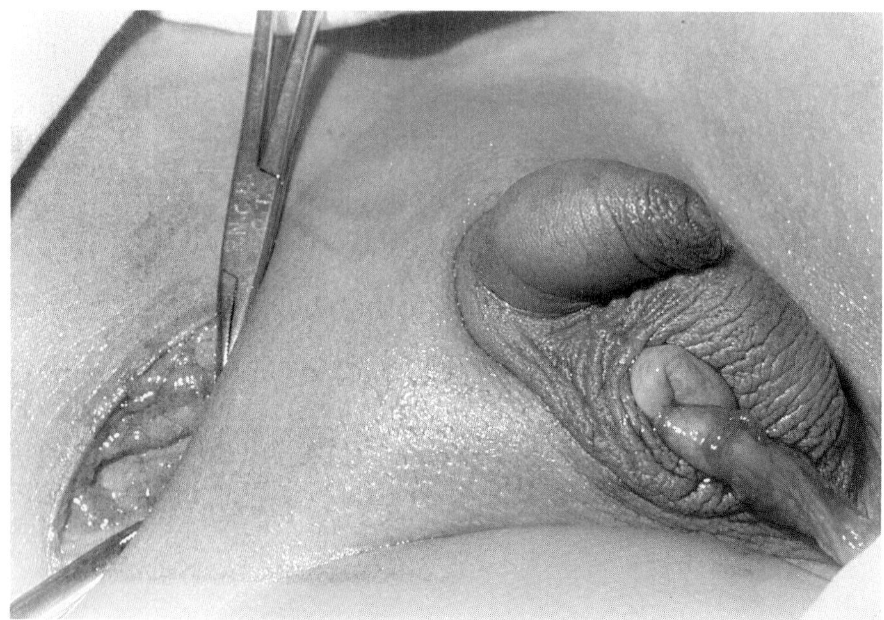

Figure 7.15 The cord (and testis) is brought into the scrotum.

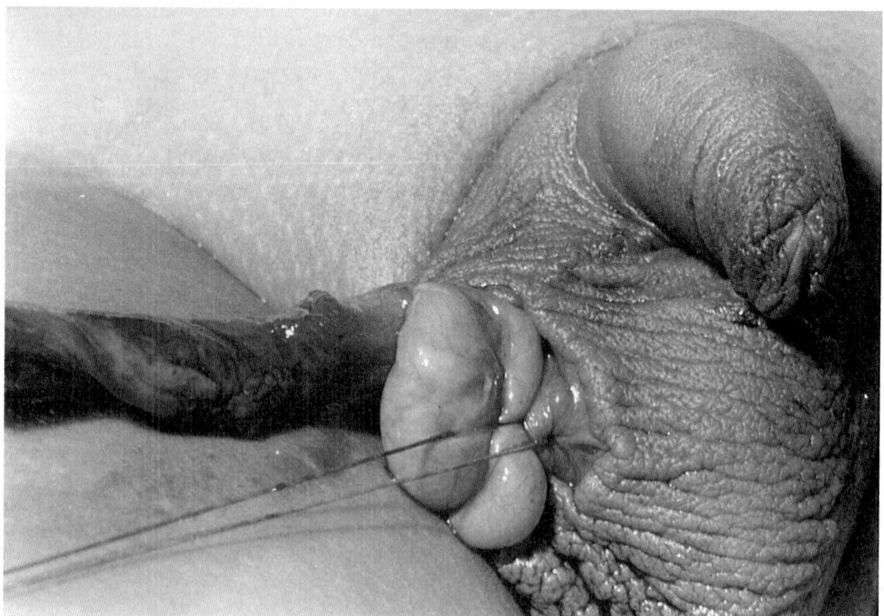

Figure 7.16 The tunica albuginea can be sutured to the midline fascia of the scrotum to prevent retraction.

a good cosmetic result. The inguinal wounds are best covered with a sterile Tegaderm or Opsite, which provides a child-proof and waterproof protection for the wound. This is removed at the post-operative review (if it has not already fallen off). The difficulty in applying such a dressing on the scrotum and the discomfort caused by its removal (particularly in the older child), means that the scrotal wound is best sprayed with a plastic skin spray, with no other dressing employed).

Local anaesthetic infiltration of both the inguinal and scrotal wounds or regional nerve blocks, ensure good analgesia in the first 4–6 hours post-operatively, the period of greatest discomfort otherwise. When the local anaesthesia wears off, paracetamol administered orally is usually adequate to control pain.

Most boys have returned to full activities within 2–4 days. The use of local anaesthesia and a light general anaesthetic allows the child to be discharged from the day surgical centre an hour or two after the operation, ideally so that he will be home and settled before the local anaesthesia has worn off. This makes transfer and transport less of an ordeal for the child (and his parents).

7.3 Unusual findings during orchidopexy

7.3.1 Testicular epididymal fusion abnormalities

In many undescended testes, particularly 'high' ones in the canal or the abdomen, the epididymis is not normally adherent to the testis.[6] Some variants of testicular–epididymal separation will cause sterility, although as long as the rete testis is intact (Figure 7.17), fertility should be normal. Concern over the implications of this anomaly has provoked some authors to recommend very careful documentation of all anatomical variants of testicular–epididymal fusion.[14] In our own institution, however, these are not sought after, and in most operations the processus vaginalis would not be opened for this purpose.

7.3.2 Ectopic tissue

Spleno-gonadal fusion (Figure 7.18) is another well-recognized entity which is probably under-reported.[15] It is occasionally seen at the time of left orchidopexy.[16] The splenic tissue should be separated from the left testis and an orchidopexy performed in the usual manner.

Ectopic renal tissue has also been described in association with an undescended testis[17,18] but must be extremely rare. A much more common finding, but one which has no significance, is ectopic adrenal cortical tissue in the spermatic cord. It appears as a 1–3 mm hard spherical and bright yellow nodule within the cord – it can be ignored.

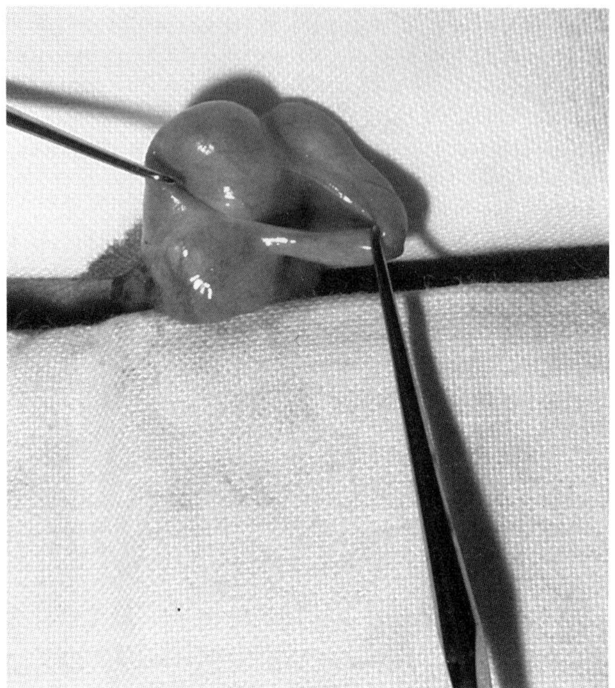

Figure 7.17 An inguinal undescended testis with separation of the epididymis except at the rete testis and the cauda. This variant would not affect fertility, as far as we know.

7.3.3 Absent vas deferens

Complete absence of the vas deferens is an occasional finding during orchidopexy. This will be seen in boys with cystic fibrosis and in some patients with related urogenital abnormalities, such as unilateral renal agenesis. Rarely, no explanation for its absence will be identifiable.

If, during orchidopexy, no vas deferens is visible during dissection of the processus vaginalis and mobilization of the cord, the following procedure is appropriate:

(1) Re-examine the cord and the processus vaginalis (by both observation and palpation) for evidence of the vas deferens.
(2) Inspect the termination of the cord to identify the epididymis and trace it proximally to locate the epididymal end of the vas deferens.
(3) Inspect the cord at the internal ring, and look for the vas deferens coursing in the extra-peritoneal space medially towards the base of the bladder.
(4) If there is still no evidence of the vas deferens, the hernial sac/processus vaginalis, once separated from the vessels and

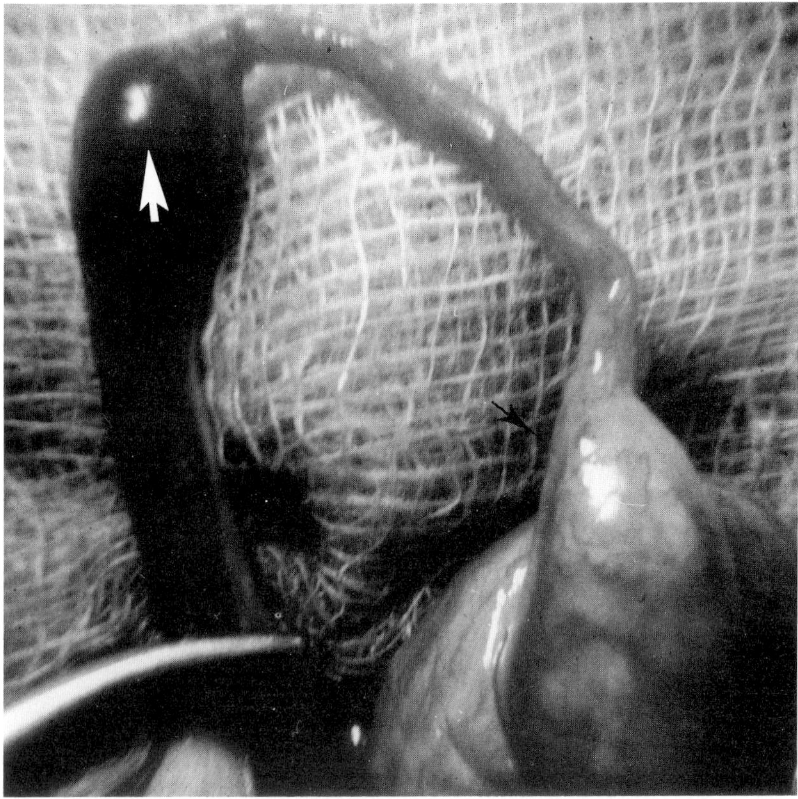

Figure 7.18 Spleno-gonadal fusion. A fibrous band connects the testis (black arrow) to the splenic tissue (white arrow).

divided, should be sent for histological examination for evidence of a vas deferens – or to confirm its absence.

(5) Post operatively, a sweat test should be obtained to exclude cystic fibrosis, the most common cause of bilateral absent vasa.

(6) A renal ultrasound may demonstrate ipsilateral renal agenesis. If the ultrasound reveals a urinary tract abnormality, completion of the screening of the urinary tract by micturating cystourethrogram would be appropriate. We have had two boys with bilateral absent vasa deferens, with normal sweat tests and unilateral absence of the kidney.

What should be done about the testis? If the testis appears normal, it would be reasonable to complete the orchidopexy, for it will fulfil its role in providing hormones, still fill the scrotum from a cosmetic point of view, and if the contralateral testis is in a similar predicament, may serve an important role in fertility, dependent on the future development of the relevant technology.

7.3.4 Persistent müllerian duct structures

A very rare syndrome that presents as undescended testis is persistent müllerian duct syndrome, in which the gene for müllerian inhibiting substance or its receptor is mutated. This leads to lack of the normal action of müllerian inhibiting substance with failure of the müllerian ducts to regress and no growth of the gubernaculum, despite normal androgen-mediated masculinization of the external genitalia and the wolffian duct. The affected child has a male external phenotype with undescended testes, and may come to surgical attention because of an inguinal hernia containing the testis. At operation, the surgeon finds one or two testes with a normal spermatic cord adjacent to an infantile uterus and fallopian tubes[19] (see Figure 2.8, page 28).

The best management of this unexpected condition is initial biopsy of the gonads and müllerian ducts to confirm the diagnosis, followed by secondary partial excision of the müllerian ducts and orchidopexy. Extreme care is required during excision to avoid damage to the vas, as it often runs in the lateral wall of the infantile uterus. Both testes may be brought down through the same inguinal canal, if required. Although there are alleged to be some men with this abnormality who are fertile, the fact that the vas deferens enters the fornix of an infantile vagina, and that the seminal vesicles are probably absent, would suggest that a normal ejaculate is unlikely.

7.4 Spermatic cord of inadequate length

7.4.1 Two-stage orchidopexy

A short spermatic cord is most likely to be a problem with testes in the inguinal canal or abdomen (Figure 7.19), where either the vas or testicular vessels may be too short to reach to the scrotum. When the testis is fully mobilized and brought as far down towards the scrotum as possible, but falls short of a satisfactory position, a second-stage orchidopexy becomes necessary. The testis is anchored as far distally as possible, and 6–18 months later, a second procedure is performed. Adhesions in the region of the testis and internal inguinal ring may make subsequent mobilization of the cord difficult and hazardous, with potential risk of injury to the testicular vessels and vas deferens which has prompted some surgeons to wrap the testis and cord in a silicone sheath.[20,21] In a series of six patients, Corkery[20] had to remove the Silastic implant in one (because of infection) and succeeded in bringing the other five testes down into the scrotum. He found marked fibrosis and 'capillary oozing' around the Silastic membrane. We have not found the Silastic sheet to be a necessary addition to the procedure.

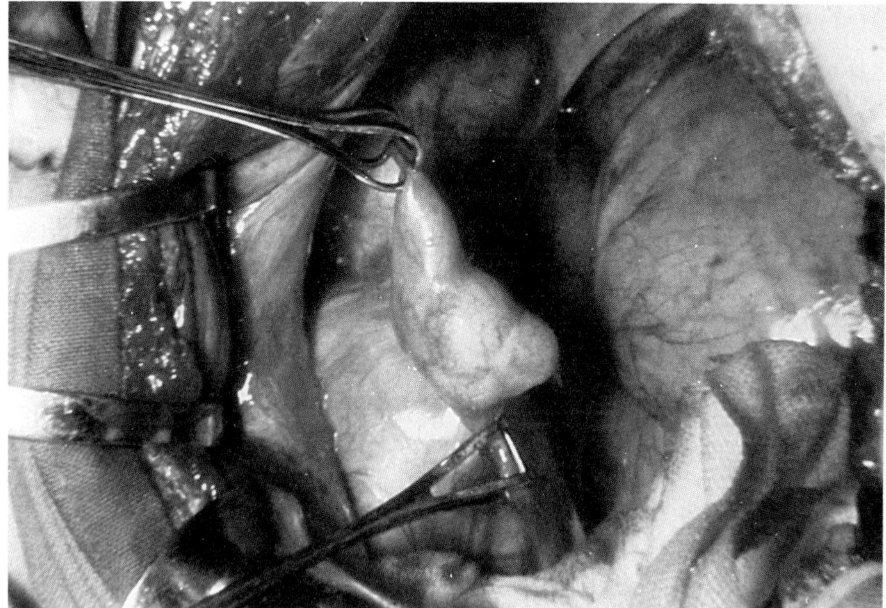

Figure 7.19 An intra-abdominal testis.

Sometimes it is evident that the vas deferens is the limiting factor preventing the testis reaching the scrotum. In this situation, the testis and cord structures can be brought down medial to the inferior epigastric vessels, thus shortening the length of vas required.

It is generally accepted that if a high retroperitoneal dissection has been done, and the testis cannot be brought into the scrotum, a staged orchidopexy is preferable to a Fowler–Stephens orchidopexy, because many of the collateral vessels which preserve the testis after testicular artery transection have been intentionally divided in the course of the retroperitoneal dissection.[22]

Not all surgeons accept that the spermatic cord lengthens after the first exploration,[23] or that the procedure is successful.[24] This is based on the observation of dense fibrous tissue surrounding the cord preventing further lengthening and that there is no demand placed on the testicular artery for it to lengthen.[23]

The success rate of staged orchidopexy has been 70–90%,[21,25,26] which is better than that achieved with the Fowler–Stephens procedure.[27] The most impressive series is that of Zer *et al.*[25] who reported 62 staged procedures: at 2–10 years, 77% were located satisfactorily in the scrotum and 65% were adequate in size; 17% had undergone partial or complete atrophy.

7.4.2 Fowler–Stephens orchidopexy

Orchidopexy involving transection of the testicular artery, was advocated in 1903 by Bevan but discouraged from 1929 because of poor results.[28]

Fowler and Stephens revived the procedure in 1959 after they demonstrated by intraoperative arteriography that collateral arterial vessels run along the vas deferens.[29] From these observations, they derived the 'Fowler–Stephens' orchidopexy. In this operation, the testicular artery is divided on the assumption that the testis will retain an adequate blood supply from the artery of the vas (or cremasteric vascular anastomoses) and that it is the testicular (spermatic, gonadal) artery which is the limiting factor in preventing an orchidopexy. The operation relies on the collateral vessels in the spermatic cord not having been disturbed; otherwise division of the testicular artery is likely to result in testicular ischaemia and atrophy.

In the series of 17 testes treated by a Fowler–Stephens orchidopexy and reported by Gibbons *et al.*[30], five atrophied, four of whom had prune belly syndrome. In 13 other patients with intra-abdominal testes, a standard Koop[31] staged orchidopexy was performed, with no atrophy occurring. Gibbons *et al.*[30] attributed their failures with the Fowler-Stephens technique to:

(1) Failure to leave a broad pedicle or tongue of vacularized visceral peritoneum overlying the vas.
(2) Attempting to salvage a scrotal placement after extensive cord mobilization and dissection.
(3) Division of the testicular artery too close to the testis, possibly compromising the vasal collateral support.
(4) Direct injury to the artery of the vas.

They add that a further contra-indication to vascular pedicle division is segmental vas atresia or a detached epididymis, as there is uncertainty that there is an adequate collateral vascular supply.

The key to the success of the Fowler–Stephens orchidopexy is prior recognition of when division of the testicular artery may be necessary, so that dissection near the critical artery to the vas can be avoided.[32] Extensive retroperitoneal dissection may also compromise the collateral vasal arterial supply,[22] and is thus a contra-indication to testicular vessel transection.

7.4.3 Two-stage Fowler–Stephens orchidopexy

The Fowler–Stephens procedure has been known for over 30 years[29] but required modification before it was to become more popular.[33] This involved deliberate staging of the procedure. As early as 1972, Engel[34] described a two-stage procedure for dividing the testicular vessels while leaving the testis *in situ*, allowing collateral vessels to be enhanced before mobilizing the testis. Ransley *et al.*[33] reported a major review of a staged Fowler–Stephens orchidopexy with promising results. In the first stage, the testicular vessels are ligated to allow the development of a collateral circulation. The subsequent orchidopexy is performed 6–12 months later, although it may be possible to reoperate as soon as 3 weeks.[33] At the second operation the artery to the vas (deferential artery) will have enlarged considerably.

This procedure is particularly useful for infants with prune belly syndrome, but may have a place in other children with impalpable testes as well. The first step, with clip ligation of the testicular vessels, has been performed successfully by laparoscopy.[35]

Division of the testicular artery too close to the testis may compromise the collateral blood supply or directly injure the artery to the vas.[30]

Traditionally, the criterion for ultimate adequacy of circulation has been the absence of postoperative testicular atrophy. Arterial flow can be demonstrated on Doppler imaging. Another method that has been described has been to use a radionuclide scrotal scan within weeks of orchidopexy involving division of the testicular vessels.[36] The adequacy of collateral blood supply can be determined during the procedure by applying an atraumatic bulldog clamp to the testicular vessels for 10 minutes and observing the general colour of the testis, and by incising the tunica albuginea and inspecting it for fresh bleeding. Only once an adequate collateral blood supply has been demonstrated are the vessels divided.

7.4.4 Microvascular anastomosis (testicular auto-transplantation)

Although transplantation of the testicular artery had been described in dogs[37] it was not until 1976 that Silber and Kelly[38] described a successful autotransplantation of an intra-abdominal testis in a child with prune belly syndrome. This development of microsurgical techniques allowed an alternative means of dealing with the high intra-abdominal testis.[39] In this procedure the testicular artery is divided and anastomosed to the inferior epigastric artery in the inguinal canal. For technical reasons this procedure is not performed until 2–4 years of age.[40] A free testicular transfer revascularization by anastomosis of the testicular vessels to the inferior epigastric vessels is now the most widely employed method.[41,42]

Bianchi[43] has reported a series of 12 testes in boys, aged 3–15 years, in which a microvascular testicular anastomosis was performed. The testicular ischaemia time ranged from 75 to 135 minutes. Arterial anastomosis failed in two (although one of these survived on the artery of the vas). The long-term results, including fertility, are unknown. In a similar series reported by Frey and Bianchi[44] the mean age at operation was 7.4 years, with an age range of 3.25–16 years.

Smaller vessels are more difficult ot anastomose, and the earlier age at which orchidopexy is performed may limit the feasibility of the technique. The skill required for the micro-technique and the equipment necessary make this method unrealistic for the majority of surgeons confronted intra-operatively with an intra-abdominal testis.[30]

Scanty results have been 'satisfactory'[45] but publication of the long-term effectiveness of the procedure is lacking. Autotransplantation of the intra-abdominal testis to the inferior epigastric vessels has been dismissed as exhibiting dramatic showmanship without being practical.[46] The two major detractions of this technique are: (1) the procedure is difficult to perform at the optimal age for orchidopexy, namely 1 year; and (2) there is no long-term post-pubertal follow-up information on its effect on fertility.

7.4.5 Post-pubertal male

In the post-pubertal male with an intra-abdominal testis, orchidectomy is appropriate on account of the poor spermatogenic potential of the gonad, and the risk of malignancy.

7.5 The unilateral impalpable testis

Before any operation, the parents should be fully informed as to the purpose of the procedure, and its possible shortcomings or complications. Following this, they would be expected to acknowledge (by signature) their informed consent for the operation to proceed: this is particularly important in the case of the boy who presents with a unilateral impalpable testis (with a normal contralateral testis). The parents should be counselled prior to surgery that there is a greater than 50% chance that the testis will be absent or be appropriately removed.[47] This makes it easier for the parents to accept the situation, should it occur, and allows the surgeon to perform an orchidectomy where appropriate, rather than to struggle to preserve a highly abnormal and potentially malignant testis, simply to protect the parents from the shock of orchidectomy. Oesch and Ransley[47] found that the impalpable testis was absent in 40% (12 out of 30); and in another five boys the testis was highly dysgenetic. Despite the fact that a unilateral impalpable testis is twice as common on the left, the outcome is similar on both sides.

In some centres, boys with unilateral impalpable testes undergo laparoscopy prior to open surgical exploration (see Chapter 6).[48] In most centres, however, including our own, surgical exploration without radiological or laparoscopic investigation is considered appropriate, and includes extension into the peritoneal cavity if the inguinal canal is empty.

In their review of 30 such patients, Oesch and Ransley[47] found that in only four patients would laparoscopy have obviated the need for surgery, i.e. in those in which a nubbin of 'vanished testis' was found at the deep inguinal ring or intra-abdominally.

7.6 Surgical management in the post-pubertal child

The management of the post-pubertal cryptorchid testis is based on an estimation of the risk of death from a germ cell testicular tumour against the risk of death from orchidectomy.[49,50] Martin and Menck in 1975[50] advocated prophylactic orchidectomy up to 50 years of age, but since then there have been improvements in survival with testicular tumours.[51] This encouraged Farrer *et al.*[49] to re-evaluate the relative risks. Based on a 0.04% incidence of germ cell tumours in cryptorchid patients, and the fact that 68% occur in those aged 15–35 years, they found the risk of surgery begins to outweigh the risk of deaths from germ cell testicular tumours at 32–34 years.

7.7 Indications for orchidectomy

The profferred indications for orchidectomy, rather than orchidopexy, for undescended testes are as follows, although the exact applications may be disputed:

(1) Unilateral cryptorchidism in postpubertal male if testis is:
   (a) Small or dysgenetic.
   (b) Very high.
   (c) Contralateral testis fully descended and normal or hypertrophied.
(2) (?)Small dysgenetic testis at any age if contralateral testis descended.
(3) (?)Inability to bring testis into scrotum.
(4) (?)Adult with cryptorchidism. From what age?

Most clinicians would accept that if the undescended testis has persisted through puberty and is small or dysgenetic with a normal or hypertrophied, fully descended contralateral testis, orchidectomy is the treatment of choice.[52] This is especially true if the undescended testis is high.

There is less agreement on whether a small or dysgenetic testis should be removed, irrespective of age, when the opposite testis is undescended.

7.8 Complications

The complications of orchidopexy are as follows:

(1) Testicular atrophy – injury to testicular vessels.
(2) Testis not fully descended:
  (a) never reached scrotum – (i) fully mobilized cord too short; (ii) inadequate mobilization.
  (b) retracted out of scrotum – (i) excessive tension on cord; (ii) inadequate fixation in scrotum.
(3) Transection of vas deferens.
(4) Haematoma – usually from cremasteric vessels.
(5) Infection – usually of scrotum.
(6) Inguinal hernia – tearing of peritoneum at internal ring.
(7) Torsion of testis (rare) – inadequate fixation.

The most significant complication of orchidopexy results from operative injury to the testicular vessels during separation of the hernial sac and mobilization of the cord.

The testicular vessels are closely applied to the processus vaginalis: inadvertent damage to the testicular artery may render the testis ischaemic and lead to its atrophy in the months following surgery. This will be evident clinically when the testis seems to 'disappear'.

There is no evidence that early orchidopexy is associated with an increased risk of vascular damage or subsequent testis atrophy[52] although such data come from paediatric surgical centres. It may well be that there is a higher attrition rate when the procedure is done at an early age by an 'adult' general surgeon, who is unlikely to use loupe magnification. Even paediatric surgeons acknowledge a 2% incidence of testicular atrophy after hernia repair (without undescended testis) in infancy.[52] The other potential case for subsequent testicular atrophy is excessive tension on the cord which compromises blood flow through the testicular artery. Atrophy of the testis is most commonly seen when abdominal testes are brought into the scrotum or when the Fowler–Stephens procedure has been employed.[52] The testis seldom becomes atrophic when brought into the scrotum without tension.

The high intracanalicular or intra-abdominal testis on a short cord may be difficult to bring down into the scrotum, and either may be fixed in the scrotum under tension (upwards retraction) or brought only as far as the neck of the scrotum – later requiring a second procedure to bring it fully into the scrotum. In the former situation, the cord structures usually elongate with time and the final position of the testis is adequate. In a few patients, however, the testis adopts a position at the neck of the scrotum and requires a repeat orchidopexy. Most commonly, post-operative testicular retraction results from inadequate retroperitoneal mobilization of the testicular artery, from failure to strip off the cremasteric muscle fibres or by failure to ligate the patent processus vaginalis.[11] Testicular retraction may occur also following hydrocele or hernia repair if the testis is not returned to the scrotum at the end of the procedure.

Failure to separate the hernial sac completely from the remainder of the cord may lead to inadvertent opening of the peritoneum at the internal ring. If this is not recognized and closed during the procedure, an inguinal hernia may become apparent in the post-operative period.

Torsion of the testis following orchidopexy is a rare event.[13,53] It would seem reasonable to expect that to open the tunica vaginalis and suture the tunica albuginea (the capsule of the testis) to the midline fascia of the scrotum during orchidopexy, might reduce this risk.

References

1. Mengel, W, Heinz HA, Sippe WG, Hecker WC. Studies on cryptorchidism: a comparison of histological findings in the germinative epithelium before and after the second year of life. *J Pediatr Surg* 1974; **9:** 445–50.
2. Yamanaka J, Baker M, Metcalfe S, Hutson JM. Serum levels of Müllerian inhibiting substance in boys with cryptorchidism. *J Pediatr Surg* 1991; **26:** 621–3.
3. Bianchi A, Squire BR. Transscrotal orchidopexy: orchidopexy revisited. *Pediatr Surg Int* 1989; **4:** 189–92.
4. Jackson MB, Gough MH, Dudley NE. Anatomical findings at orchidopexy. *Br J Urol* 1987; **59:** 568–71.
5. Schapiro SR, Bodai BI. Current concepts of the undescended testis. *Surg Gynecol Obstet* 1978; **147:** 617.
6. Marshall FF. Anomalies associated with cryptorchidism. *Urol Clin N Am* 1982; **9:** 339–47.
7. Scorer CG. The descent of the testis. *Arch Dis Child* 1964; **39:** 605–9.
8. Heath AL, Man DW, Eckstein HB. Epididymal abnormalities associated with maldescent of the testis. *J Pediatr Surg* 1984; **19:** 47–9.
9. Redman JF. Intermittent cryptorchidism: a sign of occult inguinal hernia in pubescent boys. *J Urol* 1985; **134:** 367–8.
10. Kaplan GW. Editorial Comment. *J Urol* 1985; **134:** 368.
11. Elder JS. The undescended testis. Hormonal and surgical management. *Surg Clin N Am* 1988; **68:** 983–1003.
12. Benson CD, Lotfi MW. The pouch technique in the surgical correction of cryptorchidism in infants and children. *Surgery* 1967; **62:** 967–73.
13. O'Shaughnessy M, Walsh TN, Given HF. Testicular torsion following orchidopexy for undescended testis. *Br J Surg* 1990; **77:** 583–5.
14. Martone A, Angelone S, Aliott A, Caccioppoli U. Abnormalities of the vas deferens and epididymis: proposal of a schematic graphic card to be recorded during orchidopexy. *Ital J Pediatr Surg* 1988; **2:** 79–80.
15. Ceccacci L, Tosi S. Splenic–gonadal fusion: case report and review of the literature. *J Urol* 1981; **126:** 558–9.
16. Lanza P, Docimo ASC. Splenic–gonadal fusion in cryptorchidism. *Eur Urol* 1987; **13:** 210–2.
17. McDougall EM, Mikhael BR, Carpenter B. Ectopic renal tissue associated with an undescended testis: a case report. *J Urol* 1986; **86:** 1018–9.
18. Jona JZ, Glicklich M, Cohen RD. Ectopic single ureter and severe renal dysplasia: an unusual presentation. *J Urol* 1979; **121:** 369–70.
19. Hutson JM, Chow CW, Ng WD. Persistent müllerian duct syndrome with transverse testicular ectopia. *Pediatr Surg Int* 1987; **2:** 191–4.

20. Corkery JJ. Staged orchiopexy – a new technique. *J Pediatr Surg* 1975; **10:** 515–8.
21. Steinhardt GF, Kroovand RL, Perlmutter AD. Orchiopexy: planned 2-stage technique. *J Urol* 1985; **133:** 434–5.
22. Kogan SJ, Houman BZ, Reda EF, Levitt SB. Orchiopexy of the high undescended testis by division of the spermatic vessels: a critical review of 38 selected transections. *J Urol* 1989; **141:** 1416–9.
23. Redman JF. The staged orchiopexy: a critical review of the literature. *J Urol* 1977; **117:** 113–4.
24. Fonkalsrud EW. Current concepts in the management of the undescended testis. *Surg Clin N Am* 1970; **50:** 847–52.
25. Zer M, Wolloch Y, Dintsman M. Staged orchiorrhaphy. Therapeutic procedure in cryptorchid testicle with a short spermatic cord. *Arch Surg* 1975; **110:** 387–90.
26. Firor HV. Two-stage orchiopexy. *Arch Surg* 1971; **102:** 598–9.
27. Snyder H McC, Duckett JW. Orchidopexy with division of spermatic vessels: review of 10 year experience (Abstract). *J Urol* 1984; **131:** 126A.
28. Bevan AD. The operation for undescended testis: a further study and report. *Ann Surg* 1929; **90:** 847–63.
29. Fowler R, Stephens FD. The role of testicular vascular anatomy in the salvage of high undescended testes. *Aust NZ J Surg* 1959; **29:** 92–106.
30. Gibbons MD, Cromie WJ, Duckett JW. Management of the abdominal undescended testicle. *J Urol* 1979; **122:** 76–9.
31. Koop CE. Technique of herniorrhaphy and orchiopexy. Section VI: Cryptorchidism. In: Bergsma D, Duckett JW, eds. *Urinary System and Malformations in Children*. New York: Alan R Liss, 1977: p.303.
32. Snyder H McC. Editorial comment. *J Urol* 1989; **141:** 1419.
33. Ransley PG, Vordermark JS, Caldamone AA, *et al*. Preliminary ligation of the gonadal vessels prior to orchiopexy for the intra-abdominal testicle: a staged Fowler–Stephens procedure. *World J Urol* 1984; **2:** 266–8.
34. Engel RE. The empty scrotum. *Med World News* 1972; 69–71.
35. Bloom DA. Two-step orchiopexy with pelviscopic clip ligation of the spermatic vessels. *J Urol* 1991; **145:** 1030–3.
36. Datta NS, Tanaka T, Zinner NR, Mishkin FS. Division of spermatic vessels in orchiopexy: radionuclide evidence of preservation of testicular circulation. *J Urol* 1977; **118:** 447–9.
37. Hodges CV, Behman AM, Attaran S. Transplantation of the internal spermatic artery: an experimental study. *J Urol* 1964; **91:** 90.
38. Silber SJ, Kelly J. Successful autotransplantation of an intra-abdominal testis to the scrotum by microvascular technique. *J Urol* 1976; **115:** 452–4.
39. O'Brien BMcC, Rao VK, MacLeod AH, Morrison WA, MacMahon RA. Microvascular testicular transfer. *Plastic Reconstruct Surg* 1983; **71:** 87–90.
40. Elder JS. Laparoscopy and Fowler–Stephens orchiopexy in the management of the impalpable testis. *Urol Clin N Am* 1989; **16:** 399–411.
41. Domini R, Lima M, Appignani A. Auto-transplantation of the testicle in children utilizing microsurgical technique. *Z Kinderchir* 1985; **40:** 351–4.
42. Shiosvilli TI. Bilateral abdominal cryptorchidism in males: auto-transplantation of the testis. *Eur Urol* 1985; **11:** 386–7.
43. Bianchi A. Microvascular orchidopexy for high undescended testes. *Br J Urol* 1984; **56:** 521–4.
44. Frey P, Bianchi A. Microvascular autotransplantation of intra-abdominal testes. *Progr Pediatr Surg* 1989; **23:** 115–25.
45. Wacksman, J, Dinner M, Nandler M. Results of testicular autotransplantation

using microvascular technique: experience with 8 intra-abdominal testes. *J Urol* 1982; **128:** 1319.

46. Duckett JW. Laparoscopy for cryptorchidism. In: *Dialogues in Pediatric Urology* (Weiss RM, ed). Pearl River, NY: William Millar, 1988; **11:** 6–7.
47. Oesch I, Ransley PG. Unilaterally impalpable testis. *Eur Urol* 1987; **13:** 324–6.
48. Guiney EJ, Corbally M, Malone PS. Laparoscopy and the management of the impalpable testis. *Br J Urol* 1985; **63:** 313–6.
49. Farrer JH, Walker AH, Rajfer J. Management of the postpubertal cryptorchid testis: a statistical review. *J Urol* 1989; **134:** 1071–6.
50. Martin DC, Menck HR. The undescended testis: management after puberty. *J Urol* 1975; **114:** 77–9.
51. Li FP, Connelly RR, Myers M. Improved survival rates among testis cancer patients in the United States. *J Am Med Assoc* 1982; **247:** 825–6.
52. King LR. Optimal treatment of children with undescended testes. *J Urol* 1984; **131:** 734–5.
53. Steinbruchel DA, Hansen MK. Testicular torsion after previous orchiopexy. *Br J Surg* 1978; **75:** 47.
54. Gross RE, Jewett TC, Jr. Surgical experiences from 1,222 operations for undescended testis. *J Am Med Assoc* 1956; **160:** 634–41.
55. Swenson O. *Pediatric Surgery*, New York: Appleton-Century-Crofts, 1958.
56. Potts WJ. *The Surgeon and the Child*. Philadelphia: WB Saunders, 1959.
57. Snyder WH, Greaney EM. Cryptorchidism. In: Mustard WT, Ravitch MM, Snyder WH, Welch KJ, Benson CD, eds. *Pediatric Surgery*. Chicago: Year Book Medical Publishers, 1969: Vol. 2, pp. 1292–1312.
58. Jones PG (ed). *Clinical Paediatric Surgery. Diagnosis and Management*. Sydney: Ure Smith, 1970.
59. Jones PG (ed). *Clinical Paediatric Surgery. Diagnosis and Management*. Oxford: Blackwell Scientific, 1976: 2nd edn.
60. Campbell JR. Undescended testes. In: Holder TM, Ashcraft KW, eds. *Pediatric Surgery*. Philadelphia: Saunders, 1980: p. 818.
61. Fonkalsrud EW, Mengel W. *The Undescended Testis*. Chicago: Year Book Medical Publishers, 1981.
62. Jones PG, Woodward AA (eds). *Clinical Paediatric Surgery. Diagnosis and Management*. Melbourne: Blackwell Scientific, 1986: 3rd edn.
63. Hutson JM, Beasley SW, Woodward AA. *Jones' Clinical Paediatric Surgery. Diagnosis and Management*. Melbourne: Blackwell Scientific, 1992: 4th edn.

8

Hormonal treatment

8.1 Historical background

The idea that hormonal treatment might be effective in undescended testis probably dates from the early part of this century, when it was first appreciated that sexual development might be controlled by hormones.[1] In 1928, urine of pregnant women was noted to contain a substance which stimulated the ovary and testis.[2,3] A few years later extracts of pregnancy urine were used to treat adolescents and young men with hypogonadism and undescended testes.[4]

In 1932, Engle[5] induced descent of the testes experimentally in the macacus monkey by administering hormone extracts from the anterior pituitary and pregnancy urine. These early studies in Germany and America led to a large number of clinical trials of hormonal extracts containing anterior pituitary hormones which demonstrated induction of testicular descent at widely varying rates.[6] Human pregnancy urine – which also contains hypothalamic gonadotrophins – was successful in inducing descent of the testes as well.[7] Hamilton and Hubert[8] even treated children with extracts of the recently synthesized androgen and demonstrated descent of the testes in some cases. However, the treatment induced precocious puberty, causing the direct use of androgens to fall into disfavour. As the years passed, purified human chorionic gonadotrophin (hCG) became available and for many years was a standard treatment for undescended testes in many parts of the world. Success rates with this substance varied enormously (0% to 90%).[9] HCG is still in use in many centres[10] but in Europe luteinizing hormone releasing hormone (LHRH) has replaced hCG treatment because it can be administered intra-nasally rather than by intra-muscular injection.

8.2 Rationale for treatment

Hormonal treatment is based on the controversial hypothesis that the hypothalamic–pituitary–gonadal axis is deficient in infants with undescended testis. Empirical evidence from the earlier studies in the 1930s led to the simplistic idea that androgen deficiency caused undescended testes, and therefore hormonal stimulation of androgen production would induce testicular descent. Androgen itself was abandoned as a form of treatment because of the side-effects of precocious puberty. However, it was believed that hCG, or LHRH, would stimulate local production of testosterone sufficient to induce descent without causing such a high elevation in serum testosterone that the unpleasant side-effects were produced. At the time, the 'deficient hypothalamic–pituitary testicular axis theory of cryptorchidism' was developing, it was not realized that testicular descent was such a complicated process as is now appreciated, and has been outlined in Chapters 2 and 3. In particular, it was not suspected that androgens might have an indirect action on the gubernaculum.

The main supportive evidence for the hypothalamic–pituitary testicular axis theory came from clinical studies of low serum testosterone levels in infants between 1 and 4 months of age when cryptorchidism was present.[11] It was presumed that low androgen levels represented primary deficiency, although it is quite likely that they represent secondary gonadal failure as a result of maldescent. Not all reports, however, showed such low serum testosterone and gonadotrophin levels in cryptorchid infants,[12] and in recent years the main supporting evidence has come from experimental studies on the oestrogen-treated fetal mouse. As mentioned in Chapter 2, this animal model showed that exogenous oestrogen inhibited androgen production in the fetal mouse – and this was thought to be responsible secondarily for undescended testes. The evidence we have presented in Chapter 2, however, discredits this theory. Instead, the evidence suggests that oestrogen acts via a non-androgenic mechanism to cause undescended testes, and that this mechanism is more likely to be due to inhibition of müllerian inhibiting substance.

The idea that local stimulation of gonadal androgens by LHRH treatment would cause descent is at odds with our own concept of how inguino-scrotal descent occurs (Figure 8.1). Our recent evidence that the genitofemoral nerve may control migration of the gubernaculum suggests that local high concentrations of androgen would have no significant effect on the gubernaculum. Further, a unilateral abnormality in one genitofemoral nerve would account for the fact that cryptorchidism is usually unilateral. By contrast, the hypothalamic–gonadal axis deficiency hypothesis does not account for unilateral maldescent.

The differentiation of the genitofemoral nerve in the fetus is likely to be an irreversible process with regard both to its peripheral pathway to the

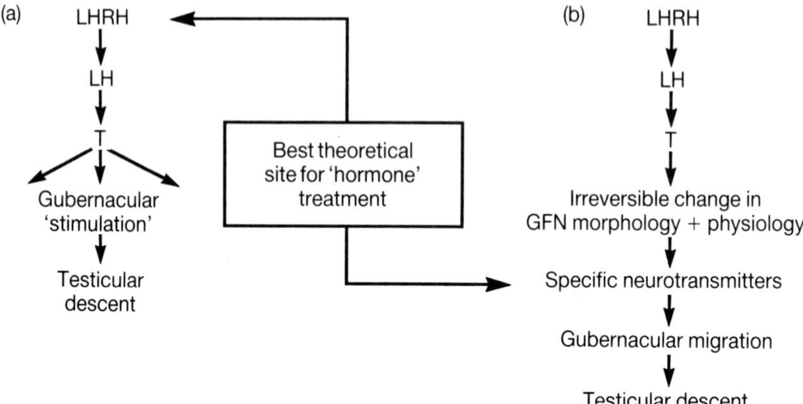

Figure 8.1 Comparison of (a) the rationale for treatment based on the hypothesis of hypothalamic–pituitary–testicular axis deficiency, where LHRH (or hCG) is administered exogenously, with (b) our own tentative hypothesis that addition of the specific neurotransmitter released by the genitofemoral nerve may be a way to stimulate testicular descent. There is little direct evidence to support this latter hypothesis at present, although it follows logically from our work on the role of the genitofemoral nerve.

inguino-scrotal region and to its potential masculinization by androgens. It would seem fanciful, therefore, to expect androgenic treatment during subsequent childhood to have any significant effect on testicular descent unless the genitofemoral nerve is normally sited and functional. Rather, it suggests that hormonal therapy for cryptorchidism should be aimed specifically at mimicking the action of the neurotransmitters released from the nerve instead of a non-specific elevation of serum testosterone. 'Ascending' testes, however, where descent has occurred postnatally, could be presumed to have normal genitofemoral anatomy and (near) normal gubernacular migration to the scrotum; the defect being (?) failure of elongation of the spermatic cord and cremaster muscle with growth: these testes would be predicted to respond well to androgenic stimulation by growth of the muscle and cord structures. In addition, retractile testes are known to respond well to hCG or LHRH since androgens need only stimulate relaxation of the cremaster muscle in these cases to produce 'descent'.

8.3 Standard regimens

A number of different administration regimens have been proposed for hCG treatment of boys with undescended testes. They range from 100 IU per kg at 4–5 day intervals for 4 weeks[13] to 1000 IU weekly for 2 weeks.[14] Christiansen *et al.* administered hCG twice a week for 3 weeks using 100 IU per kg up to a maximum of 1500 IU. Saggese *et al.*[14] gave FSH (simultaneously with hCG) in a dose of 75 IU weekly for 6 weeks, but found that the addition of FSH made little appreciable difference to the results.

The dose regimen for LHRH is reasonably standardized: it is usually given in a spray with 100 mg in each nostril six times a day for 4 weeks. Alternative regimens administer 200 mg to each nostril three times a day.[15–20] Apart from intra-nasal spray, the other method of LHRH administration tried was pulsatile intravenous injection using a portable syringe pump.[21] LHRH was administered in doses of 10–100 mg per day given in a 3 minute pulse every hour for 3–19 weeks. A battery-operated programmable syringe driver was used with a daily insertion of the scalp vein needle into a vein on the anterior abdominal wall. The needle was changed daily by the parents. This complex regimen was developed in an attempt to simulate natural hypothalamic secretion rather than to follow the pharmacological approach used by others.[21] It has since been abandoned because this degree of intervention was not well tolerated by the patients and the results were poor.

8.4 Does hormonal treatment work?

The results of hCG treatment have been variable, and appear to depend very much on the initial position of the testis. The success rate of treatment has ranged from 25% to 55%.[22,23]

The factors associated with successful hormone treatment are:

(1) Initial low testicular position (i.e. scrotal entrance).
(2) Over 4 years of age.
(3) Bilateral undescended testes.
(4) Retractile testes.

When used for retractile testes, the success rate is 95–100%.[4,15] By contrast, impalpable testes have a very low success rate. Hormone treatment is less successful in infants than in older children, and there is a significant risk of relapse following treatment, with reascent of the testes in 10–30%.[24] The factors that predict outcome of hCG treatment are shown in Table 8.1.

Christiansen *et al.*[25] had a 25% success rate with hCG in achieving complete descent of the testis. In a further 25%, the treatment improved the position of the testis. These patients all had bilateral undescended testes initially. On the other hand, in unilateral undescended testes, only 14% of boys had successful treatment. Garagorri *et al.*[26] found that infants had a lower success rate than children more than 3–4 years of age. Forest *et al.*[13] had an overall success rate with hCG treatment of 40.5%. However, they had a classification which included testes that were apparently inside the inguinal canal, but most surgeons would agree with Denis Browne[27] that intra-canalicular testes are very difficult or impossible to palpate.

Table 8.1 'Success' rates reported with hCG treatment

Authors	Number of patients	UDTs	Complete descent(%)
Bergada[32]	1200	–	30–40
Bierich[23]	–	612	55
Canlorbe *et al.*[33]	130	–	39
Dickerman *et al*[22].	128	–	55
Forest *et al.*[34]	–	558	36
Knorr[24]	–	574	52
Pagliano–Sassi[35]	–	115	54

Reproduced with permission from Reference 10.
UDTs = Undescended testes.

In a randomized, double-blind study comparing hCG and LHRH, Rajfer *et al.*[15] found that 6% of boys treated with hCG had descended testes compared with 19% of those treated with LHRH. They excluded children who had definite retractile testes; however, these children still received treatment and had a very high success rate. They concluded that hormonal therapy with either LHRH or hCG was ineffective in promoting testicular descent in boys with truly undescended testes. However, short-term treatment with hCG was effective in producing descent of retractile testis. They speculated that the discrepancies in the literature in apparent efficacy of hormonal therapy may be caused by inclusion in many studies of a variable proportion of patients with retractile testes.

In a double-blind placebo-controlled study of LHRH nasal spray, de Muinck Keizer-Schrama *et al.*[12] had a 9% success rate with LHRH therapy compared with 8% in placebo-treated boys. After a second course of LHRH they noted that a few more children responded to treatment giving an overall success rate for LHRH nasal spray of 18% (Figure 8.2). Their success rate was lowest in the youngest children and highest in the older age groups, and much greater in those testes that were closest to the scrotum. The authors measured the hormonal response to LHRH therapy, and found no evidence of a deficiency of the hypothalamic–pituitary axis, or any deficiency in Leydig cell function. They concluded that LHRH nasal spray was not useful for impalpable testes but may have a small role in those children with testes near the neck of the scrotum. De Muinck Keizer-Schrama[10] has reviewed the literature on hormone treatment for undescended testes using LHRH nasal spray, and found the reported success rates varied from 9% (her own results) to 78% (Table 8.2).

8.5 Possible benefits of hormonal treatment

The advantage of hormonal therapy would appear to be in distinguishing undescended testes from retractile testes. Retractile testes respond by

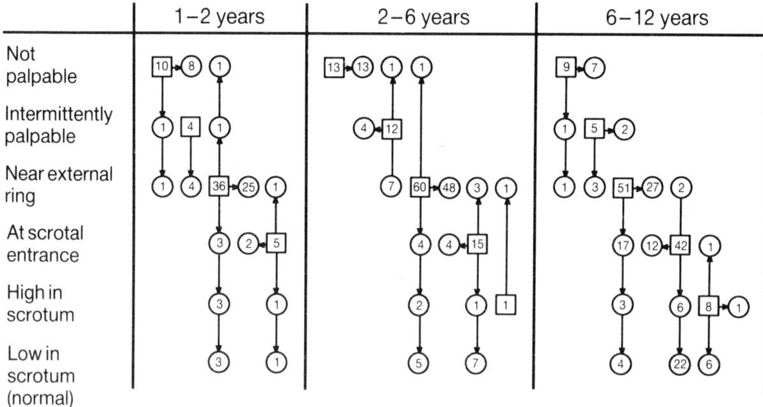

Figure 8.2 The most caudal position of the testis (indicated by the number of testes) before (□) and after (O) LHRH treatment intranasally (excluding placebo descents). These results are from the double-blind, placebo-controlled trial of LHRH nasal spray performed by de Muinck Keizer-Schrama *et al.*,[12] and are reproduced with permission of authors and publisher.

descent almost uniformly, in stark contrast to ectopic or impalpable testes that almost never respond to treatment. Many authors have suggested, therefore, that hormonal therapy could be used to distinguish retractile testes from truly undescended testes.

Hadziselimovic[28] has suggested that hormonal therapy may have a further role in stimulating testicular physiology to restore the normal function of the testes after surgery. He biopsied 15 of 31 testes that failed to descend in response to hormone treatment and required orchidopexy.[28] LHRH therapy caused a marked increase in the size of the Leydig cells and in their content of endoplasmic reticulum, suggesting a recruitment of precursor Leydig cells from fibroblasts. In addition, he has suggested that the number of germ cells per tubule may be increased after LHRH therapy independent of the need for surgical treatment. In other words, he has proposed that even though surgery may be required to relocate the undescended testes into the scrotum, hormone treatment may be needed in addition to stimulate normal germ cell maturation. Insufficient work has been done so far on the effect of hormone treatment on fertility, making it difficult at present to evaluate this hypothesis. However, the idea that the position of the testes and the physiology of the testes may need separate treatment needs careful consideration.

8.6 Why hormonal treatment fails

In a collaborative study with de Muinck Keizer-Schrama, Hazebroek[29] investigated the anatomical reasons for failure of LHRH hormonal therapy.

Table 8.2 Success rates reported for LHRH nasal spray treatment

Reference	LHRH nasal spray			Patients		Number of testes	Percentage of complete descent	
	Daily dose	Duration (weeks)	+/−	No.	Age (years)		Patients	Testes
Illig *et al.*[36]	6×200	4	+	46	1–12	61		38
Bertelsen *et al.*[37]	6×200	4	+	23	5–12	34	26	24
Hagberg and Westphal[38]	6×100	4	+	47	2–10	61		28
Karpe *et al.*[20]	6×200	4	+	25	3–8	25	20	20
Wit *et al.*[39]	3×400	4	+	26	1–12	35		17
De Muinck Keizer-Schrama *et al.*[19]	3×400	4	+	121	1–13	151	9	9
Happ *et al.*[18]	6×200	1-10	−	25	1–11	36		64
Pirazzoli *et al.*[16]	6×200	1	−	9	5–12	9	22	22
	6×500	1	−	13	5–12	13	39	39
Zabransky[40]	6×200	4	−	40	1–14	50		78
Cacciari *et al.*[41]	6×200	1	−	23	3–12	23	22	22
	2×500	1	−	24	3–12	24	38	38
Hagberg and Westphal[37]	3×400	4	−	49	2–10	56		61
Hadziselimovic *et al.*[42]	3×400	4	−	60	$^{10}/_{12}$–14	81		62
Borkenstein *et al.*[43]	3×400	4	−	53	1.2–12	68	49	57
Van der Meijden *et al.*[44]	6×200	4	−	29	2–12	39		13
Schwarz *et al.*[45]	3×400	4	−	119	1–12	171		37
De Muinck Keizer-Schrama *et al.*[12]	3×400	2×4	−	227	1–13	271		18
Job *et al.*[46]	3×400	4	−	39	1–6	46		
	2×400	4–12*	−	54	2–6	74		21

\+ = Placebo-controlled study; − = open study.
*On alternate day
Reproduced with permission from Reference 10.

After two courses of LHRH nasal spray, 48 out of 281 testes (18%) in 237 prepubertal boys had undergone full descent into the scrotum. Of the unsuccessfully treated boys, 170 subsequently had orchidopexy for 196 persistently undescended testes. At operation, anatomical abnormalities that were believed to account for the failure of hormone treatment were found in 80% of children. Hazebroek found the most common abnormality to be failure of the processus vaginalis to extend beyond the level of the pubic bone. In addition, these testes were often associated with major epididymal abnormalities or a persistence of a patent processus vaginalis. In a small number of children, the surgeon noted an abnormal attachment of Scarpa's fascia obliterating the entrance to the scrotum. This study is consistent with many others which together suggest that in ectopic testicular descent or in the testis in which a presumed mechanical abnormality is present (e.g. obstruction at the neck of the scrotum) the response to hormone treatment is poor.

The failure of hormonal therapy except in retractile testes is consistent with what we now know of the aetiology of normal testicular descent. Much of the early work on hormonal therapy was based on Engle's original animal studies in the immature macaque monkey.[5] His ability to induce premature descent of the testis in the macaque monkey provided an experimental basis for many subsequent studies. Interestingly the macaque monkey is a very unusual animal, in that the testes descend fully into the scrotum before birth, and then re-ascend out of the scrotum and remain in the groin until the onset of puberty.[30] However, at the time of Engle's experimental study, this curious fact about the macaque monkey was not appreciated. Therefore, hormonal treatment of the immature macaque monkey induced 'descent' by initiating precocious puberty. In effect, it caused descent of a naturally retractile testis. Indeed, many authors have postulated that successful hormone treatment is caused by relaxation of the cremaster muscle, allowing the testes to descend to an apparently lower level.[20,31]

Further reasons for failure of hormonal therapy follow logically from our current hypothesis of inguino-scrotal descent (see Chapter 3). As shown in Figure 8.1, it is our postulate that androgens act indirectly on gubernacular migration via the genitofemoral nerve, and that this process is likely to be irreversible. The genitofemoral nerve is probably 'masculinized' in the middle trimester of pregnancy, with the male nerve becoming larger and containing significantly greater amounts of calcitonin gene-related peptide (and possibly other transmitters) than in the female. Hormonal stimulation postnatally is unlikely to reverse this morphological differentiation. If the failure of descent has been caused by an anatomical abnormality of the genitofemoral nerve (e.g. failure of the peripheral axons to reach the lower scrotum) hormonal therapy stimulating androgen production would never be expected to cause testicular descent. By contrast, administration of the neurotransmitters released naturally by the genitofemoral nerve (e.g. calcitonin gene-related peptide) may in the future have a role in the non-surgical treatment of undescended testis.

8.7 Conclusions

Hormone treatment for undescended testes has been tried for around 60 years with very limited success. Initial enthusiastic reports, first with androgens, then hCG and finally LHRH, have been replaced by subsequent poor results. Even the original study by Engle,[5] which stimulated so much clinical experimentation, has turned out to be erroneous. It is now well established that hCG and LHRH therapy have no significant place in the treatment of true cryptorchidism. Their potential role in the management of ascending or retractile testes, however, remains controversial. They may become useful ways to diagnose these apparently acquired anomalies.

LHRH treatment may be important as an adjunct to surgery to stimulate germ cell maturation, and hence reverse the potential infertility of maldescended testes after operation. This is a new and exciting concept that needs further experimental exploration before it can be considered a serious therapeutic option. It does, however, offer great promise as a way to improve the long-term results.

At present, hormone treatment should be reserved for those institutions carrying out controlled trials, and cannot be recommended for general use. In some older children, where there is a strong likelihood of the high testis being 'retractile' or 'ascending', hormone therapy may confirm the diagnosis and avoid surgery. LHRH treatment would seem superior to hCG administration, if only because a series of painful injections can be avoided.

References

1. Lillie FR. The theory of the freemartin. *Science* 1916; **43:** 611.
2. Ascheim S, Zondek B. Die schwanger schaftsdiagnose aus dem harn durch nachweis des hypophysenvorderlappenhormons: I Grundlagen und technik der methode. *Klin Wochenschr* 1928; **30:** 1404–11.
3. Ascheim S, Zondek B. Die schwange schaftsdiagnose aus dem harn durch nachweis des hypophysenvorderlappenhormons: II Praktische und theoretische ergebnisse aus den harnuntersuchungen. *Klin Wochenschr* 1928; **31:** 1453–57.
4. Schapiro B. Kann man mit hypophysenvorderlappen den unterentwickelten männlichen genitalapparat beim menschen zum wachstum anregen? *Dtsch Med Wochenschr* 1930; **56:** 1605–7.
5. Engle ET. Experimentally induced descent of testis in the Macacus monkey

by hormones from anterior pituitary and pregnancy urine. *Endocrinology* 1932; **16:** 513–20.

6. Thompson WO, Bevan AD, Heckel NJ, *et al*. The treatment of undescended testes with anterior pituitary-like substance. *Endocrinology* 1937; **21:** 220–9.
7. Bigler JA, Hardy LM, Scott HV. Cryptorchidism treated with gonadotropic principle. *Am J Dis Child* 1938; **55:** 273–94.
8. Hamilton JB, Hubert G. Effect of synthetic male hormone substance on descent of testicles in human cryptorchidism. *Proc Soc Exp Biol Med* 1938; **39:** 4.
9. Deming CL. The evolution of hormonal therapy in cryptorchidism. *J Urol* 1952; **68:** 354–7.
10. De Muinck Keizer-Schrama SMPF. Hormonal treatment of cryptorchidism. *Horm Res* 1988; **30:** 178–86.
11. Job JC, Toublanc JE, Chaussain JL, Gendrel D, Garnier P, Roger M. Endocrine and immunological findings in cryptorchid infants. *Horm Res* 1988; **30:** 167–72.
12. De Muinck Keizer-Schrama SMPF, Hazebroek FWJ. *The Treatment of Cryptorchidism. Why, How, When. Clinical Studies in Prepubertal Boys*. Erasmus University, Rotterdam: Theses. 1986.
13. Forest MG, David M, David L, Chatelain PG, Francois R, Bertrand J. Undescended testis: comparison of two protocols of treatment with human chorionic gonadotropin. *Horm Res* 1988; **30:** 198–206.
14. Saggese G, Ghirri P, Gabrielli S, Cosenza GCM. Hormonal therapy for cryptorchidism with a combination of human chorionic gonadotropin and follicle-stimulating hormone. *Am J Dis Child* 1989; **143:** 980–2.
15. Rajfer J, Handelsman DJ, Swerdloff RS, *et al*. Hormonal therapy of cryptorchidism. A randomised, double-blind study comparing human chorionic gonadotropin and gonadotropin-releasing hormone. *N Engl J Med* 1986; **314:** 466–70.
16. Pirazzoli P, Zappulla F, Bernardi F, *et al*. Luteinizing hormone-releasing hormone nasal spray as therapy for undescended testicle. *Arch Dis Child* 1978; **53:** 235–8.
17. Wit JM, Delemarre-Van De Waal HA, Bax NMA, Van Den Brande JL. Effect of LHRH treatment on testicular descent and hormonal response in cryptorchidism. *Clin Endocrinol* 1986; **24:** 539–48.
18. Happ J, Kollmann F, Krawehl C, *et al*. Treatment of cryptorchidism with pernasal gonadotropin-releasing hormone therapy. *Fertil Steril* 1978; **29:** 546–51.
19. De Muinck Keizer-Schrama SMPF, Hazebroek FWJ, Matroos AW, Drop SLS, Molenaar JC, Visser HKA. Double-blind, placebo-controlled study of luteinizing-hormone-releasing-hormone nasal spray in treatment of undescended testes. *Lancet* 1986; **i:** 876–80.
20. Karpe B, Eneroth P, Ritzen EM. LHRH treatment in unilateral cryptorchidism: effect on testicular descent and hormonal response. *J Pediatr* 1983; **103:** 892–7.
21. Keogh EJ, Mackellar A, Mallal SA, *et al*. Treatment of cryptorchidism with pulsatile luteinizing hormone-releasing hormone (LH-RH). *J Pediatr Surg* 1983; **18:** 282–3.
22. Dickerman Z, Bauman B, Sandovsky U, *et al*. HCG treatment in cryptorchidism. *Andrologia* 1983; **16:** 542–7.
23. Bierich JR. Treatment by human chorionic gonadotrophin in maldescended testes. In: Bierich JR, Rager K, Ranke MB, eds. *Maldescensus testis*, Munich: Urban & Schwarzenberg, 1977: pp. 101–9.

24. Knorr D. Diagnose und therapie der deszensusstorungen des hodens. *Padiatr Prax* 1970; **9:** 299–304.
24. Bierich JR. Clinical treatment of maldescensus testis. In: Cryptorchidism (Bierich JR, Giarola A, eds). London, Academic Press, 1979: pp. 375–89.
25. Christiansen P, Müller J, Buhl S, *et al.* Treatment of cryptorchidism with human chorionic gonadotropin or gonadotropin releasing hormone. *Horm Res* 1988; **30:** 187–92.
26. Garagorri J-M, Job J-C, Canlorbe P, Chaussain J-L. Results of early treatment of cryptorchidism with human chorionic gonadotropin. *J Pediatr* 1982; **101:** 923–7.
27. Browne D. The diagnosis of undescended testicle. *Br Med J* 1938; **ii:** 168.
28. Hadziselimovic F. Hormonal treatment of the undescended testis. *J Pediatr Endocrinol* 1987; **2:** 1–5.
29. Hazebroek FWJ, De Muinck Keizer-Schrama SMPF, Van Maarschalkerweerd M, Visser HKA, Molenaar JC. Why luteinizing-hormone-releasing-hormone nasal spray will not replace orchidopexy in the treatment of boys with undescended testes. *J Pediatr Surg* 1987; **22:** 1177–82.
30. Kinzey WG. Male reproductive system and spermatogenesis. In: Hafez ESF, ed. *Comparative Reproduction of Non-Human Primates*. Springfield IL: Charles C Thomas, 1971: p. 85.
31. Karpe B. Prognosis of hormonal treatment of undescended testis related to testicular position at birth. *Pediatr Surg Int* 1991; **6:** 221–2.
32. Bergada C. Clinical treatment of cryptorchidism. In: Bierich JR, Giarola A eds. *Cryptorchidism*. London: Academic Press 1979: pp. 367–74.
33. Canlorbe P, La Clyde JP, Toublanc JE, *et al.* Results of treatment with hCG in cryptorchidism. *Pediatr Adolesc Endocrinol* 1979; **6:** 167–72.
34. Forest MG, David M, Francois R. Treatment of cryptorchidism with human chorionic gonadotropin (hCG): a 15 year experience. *Belg Ver Kindergenessk* 1985; **17:** 45–64.
35. Pagliano-Sassi L. Significance and results of medical treatment in cryptorchidism. In: Bierich JR, Giarola A, eds. *Cryptorchidism*. London: Academic Press, 1979: pp. 435–40.
36. Illig R, Exner GU, Kollmann F, *et al.* Treatment of cryptorchidism by intranasal synthetic luteinizing-hormone releasing hormone. Results of a collaborative double-blind study. *Lancet* 1977; **ii:** 518–20.
37. Bertelsen A, Skakkebaek NE, Mauritzen K, *et al.* Intranasalt gonadotropin frigorende hormon (LH-RH) som behandling ved retentio testis. *Ugeskr Laeger* 1981; **143:** 1595–7.
38. Hagberg S, Westphal O. Treatment of undescended testes with intranasal application of synthetic LHRH. *Eur J Pediatr* k1982; **139:** 285–8.
39. Wit JM, Delemarre-Van De Waal HA, Jansen M, *et al.* Resultaten van intransale toediening van synthetisch LHRH wegens niet ingedaalde testes. *Ned Tijdschr Geneeskd* 1985; **129:** 300–4.
40. Zabransky S. LH-RH Nasalspray (Kryptocur) ein neuer Aspekt in der hormonellen Behandlung des Hodenhoschstandes. *Kin Padiatr* 1981; **193:** 382–4.
40. Hadziselimovic F, Girard J, Herzog B, *et al.* Hormonal treatment of cryptorchidism. *Horm Res* 1982; **16:** 188–92.
40. Cacciari E, Frejaville E, Becca A. Treatment of cryptorchidism by intranasal synthetic LH-RH and its analogue *D*-Ser(TBU)^{6}-LHRH-EA^{10}. *Eur J Pediatr* 1982; **139:** 280–4.
41. Borkenstein M, Zobel V, Von der Ohe M. Three times daily intranasal LHRH application for treatment of cryptorchidism (abstract 83) *Pediatr Res* 1983; **18:** 115.

44. Van der Meijden APM, Schreinemachers LMH, Janknegt RA. Intransale toediening LH-RH voor de behandeling van de niet ingedaalde testis. *Ned Tijdschr Geneeskd* 1984; **129:** 992–6.
45. Schwarz HP, Aebi S, Perisic M. Success and relapse rate after treatment of cryptorchidism with intranasal LHRH. *Acta Paediatr Scand* 1985; **74:** 274–80.
46. Job JC, Joab N, Safar A, *et al.* Effets de la gonadoliberine (LHRH) par voie nasale chez les enfants cryptorchides de la 6 ans. *Arch Fr Pediatr* 1987; **44:** 91–5.

9

Results of treatment

9.1 Criteria of assessment

The results of treatment of undescended testes can be assessed at several different levels. In some boys the cosmetic appearance will be the important factor, while for others the potential for fertility is of prime importance. The risk of malignancy during young adult years is less critical initially, but becomes more important with age. At present it is not known whether the good cosmetic results will be matched by good subsequent fertility and lower risk of malignancy, because the lag time for assessment of these latter features is up to 20–40 years. The timing and method of treatment has changed so rapidly in recent years it is too soon to assess the long-term repercussions of these changes.

9.2 Cosmetic result

Surgical correction of an undescended testis will result in an intrascrotal testis of reasonable size in a very high percentage of children. Adamsen and Bornesson[1] in a review of 135 testes in 121 boys operated on at about 6 years, found that 87% of the testes were intrascrotal in long-term follow-up. Success rates in most series are higher for testes which are beyond the inguinal canal. On the other hand, testes in the canal or in the abdomen have a higher incidence of persisting abnormality following orchidopexy, mainly failure of the testes to reach the scrotum or inadequate growth or atrophy of the intra-scrotal testes. Total infarction of the testis is a well-recognized entity which occurs in approximately 3% of all patients with an impalpable undescended testis. In a further 15–20% of patients, the high intra-abdominal testis will become atrophic or need excision following failed orchidopexy. Fortunately, the intra-abdominal testis is relatively rare, representing no more than 10–15% of the total number of children with undescended testes.

Where orchidopexy has failed to bring the testis fully into the scrotum, a second operation 6–18 months later very often will be successful (see Chapter 7). However, there is a significant attrition rate of these testes with progressive atrophy occurring.

In many long-term follow-up studies, the size of the testis has been documented. In most series, testicular volume is found to be slightly lower than normal in adults following orchidopexy in childhood. Decrease in testicular volume is usually more marked in those men with a past history of bilateral orchidopexy.[2,3] There is a high incidence of secondary atrophy when orchidopexy is combined with herniotomy in infants who have presented with a strangulated hernia. The difficult dissection required in many infants with a large inguinal hernia appears to compromise the testicular vessels much more often than during routine orchidopexy, particularly if not performed by an experienced paediatric surgeon.

The risk of testicular atrophy after surgery has become an important point for debate recently with the lowering of the recommended age for surgery. A study that specifically addresses this issue, therefore, is a welcome addition to the literature.[4] These authors performed a retrospective study of infants undergoing orchidopexy to see if the risk of atrophy increased with decreasing age at operation, since paediatric surgeons are uncertain how to weigh up biological risk (of dysplasia) versus operative risk (causing atrophy). Many authors believe that although testicular dysplasia increases with age (particularly after age 2), the risk of atrophy is greater in infants because of their smaller and more delicate testicular vessels (Figure 9.1).[5,6]

Wilson-Storey *et al.*[4] compared 100 infants who had orchidopexy before their second birthday with 100 toddlers or older children undergoing surgery after their second birthday. By analysis of the hospital records and follow-up, they found that 5% of the testes became atrophic in each group, showing that with standard paediatric surgical techniques, the risk of operative damage is not related to age.

9.3 Fertility

9.3.1 Human follow-up studies

The prognosis for fertility is compromised in some men because of a primary abnormality of the testis or epididymis.[7–9] Testes which have a primary hormonal or structural abnormality, and are arrested in the line of normal descent, may have reduced potential for fertility even after treatment. The exact extent of these problems cannot be ascertained directly, because of the difficulty of correlating testicular histology in

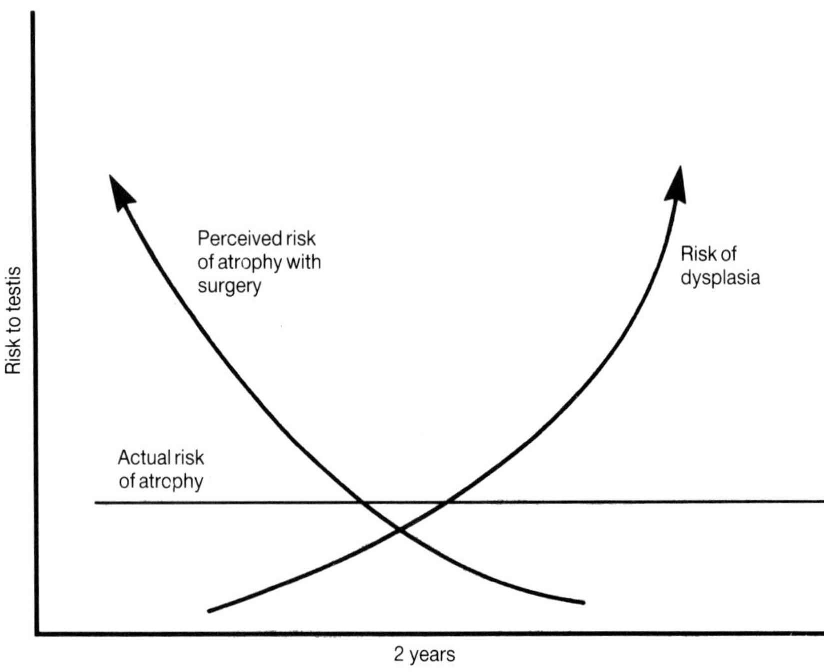

Figure 9.1 The risk of testicular atrophy is commonly thought to be greater in smaller boys, while the risk of secondary testicular dysplasia increases with age. This dilemma has made selection of the optimal time for surgery difficult and controversial. Wilson-Storey *et al.*[4] suggest that the risk of atrophy is not greater in small infants which, if confirmed, would simplify decisions about timing.

childhood with subsequent spermatogenesis during adult life. In addition, those testes with significant testicular-epididymal separation and those testes with occlusion or other abnormalities of the proximal vas deferens would not be expected to have normal fertility, even after treatment. These abnormalities, being more common in the intra-abdominal testes, may account – at least in part – for the higher incidence of infertility, despite surgery, in this small group.

Those testes initially located beyond the inguinal canal in the groin or neck of the scrotum have a good prognosis for fertility, according to most authors (Table 9.1). Puri and O'Donnell[5] performed semen analysis in 142 men who had previously had an orchidopexy between 7 and 13 years of age. There were 119 unilateral and 23 bilateral undescended testes. Using standard criteria (WHO) of semen analysis they found that the fertility potential was directly proportional to the original position of the testis. Those testes that were closest to the scrotum initially had the highest fertility potential. Testes located within the canal or the abdominal cavity were associated with azospermia. Puri and O'Donnell[5] are criticized by Tamhne and Williams[10] for only performing semen analysis on 142 of

Table 9.1 Prognosis for fertility in undescended testes after orchidopexy

Authors	No. of patients	Age at operation (years)	Fertility test	Percentage 'fertile'	
				Unilateral	Bilateral
Cendron *et al.*[12]	40	7	Paternity	87	33
Singh *et al.*[13]			Needle cytology	87	43
Werder *et al.*[5]	48	11	Semen analysis	57	14
Singer *et al.*[14]	25	6.2	Semen analysis	70	40
Puri and O'Donnell[5]	142	7–13	Semen analysis	74	30
Atkinson *et al.*[11]	40	9	Paternity	81	33

329 eligible subjects. They make the point that interpretation of semen analysis results is difficult because an equivalent 'normal' population is not available. Finally, they doubt Puri and O'Donnell's assertion that orchidopexy in younger children is more difficult or has a higher rate of complications.

In a review of 58 testes from 40 patients operated between 1939 and 1962 Atkinson *et al.*[11] found a paternity rate of 81% in those men with a past history of unilateral undescended testes, compared with a paternity rate of 33% in bilateral cases. These men had had an operation at an average age of 9 years and were investigated at 28 years. The testes were in the normal position in 86% and were a normal size in 75%. The androgen levels were normal in 90% of men, but 20% had increased serum levels of LH and 15% had increased levels of FSH.

Cendron *et al.*[12] reviewed 40 patients operated on between 1950 and 1960, where a testicular biopsy had been taken at the time of the original operation. The mean age of operation on these children was 7 years. There was an 87% paternity rate in those men with a unilateral abnormality, compared with 33% in those with bilateral undescended testes. Oligospermia was present in 16 of the 40 patients, but this was not predictive of their paternity status. They found the histological criteria on the original biopsy correlated closely with their subsequent paternity status. In a similar study Singh *et al.*[13] followed 22 men operated on between 1969 and 1979. They found a fertility potential (as measured on fine needle aspiration cytology) of 87% in unilateral cases, compared with 43% in bilateral cases. Semen analysis and testicular biopsy criteria correlated closely with their results on fine needle aspiration. They recommended this as a method of assessing likely fertility in childhood or adolescence, since it can be done readily without anaesthesia.

Werder *et al.*[3] looked at 48 men operated on at 11 years of age, between 1960 and 1961. Their age at investigation was approximately 24 years. Semen analysis was performed on 37 of these men, and six had azospermia, all of whom had a history of bilateral orchidopexy. Five had severe oligospermia and 10 had moderate oligospermia. Serum gonadotrophin levels were elevated in those men with a past history of bilateral undescended testis. Singer *et al.*[14] looked at 25 men aged between 16 and 20 who had been operated on at the mean age of 6.2 years. Their androgen, LH and prolactin levels were all within the normal range but there was a slightly elevated serum FSH level. They examined cell-mediated immunity against semen samples and found auto-antibodies against semen in 80% of those with a history of bilateral undescended testis and 45% of those with unilateral undescended testis. They speculated that secondary degeneration of the undescended testis leads to unmasking of sperm antigens, leading to the production of a cell-mediated auto-immune reaction. This immune response could lead to inhibition of sperm development in both testes, including the contralateral descended testes. Similar phenomena have been observed in adult men with a history of torsion of the testis in adolescence. It is believed that torsion leading to ischaemia damages the blood-testis barrier, exposing germ cell antigens to the immune system. Similar mechanisms are likely to occur in undescended testes where degeneration occurs.

Fertility in men after childhood orchidopexy has been assessed by comparing their age at the birth of their first child with the normal population of different parts of Scotland.[15] They were unable to show a significant effect of early operation except when the surgery was delayed beyond 18 years of age, where some delay in becoming a parent was observed. The age of orchidopexy, however, was skewed towards late childhood and early adolescence, as only one patient was included where orchidopexy had been performed before 6 years of age. Their study suffers, therefore, from showing results from a previous generation that unfortunately do not address the current issues, such as the results of surgery in infancy.

An extensive literature review of the effect of treatment has not demonstrated any significant improvement in fertility with early operation within the range of 4 to 14 years.[16] Unfortunately, however, only 4 out of 27 papers reviewed were published in the 1980s, and most of the ten reports published before 1970 describe the outcome of operations done on adolescents prior to the 1950s. As our knowledge and style of management have changed so much since then, it is impossible to compare these with what might be the results of current treatment. All that these studies tell us for certain is that subsequent fertility is poor when operation is performed in late childhood or early adolescence: they do not address the effect of surgery in infancy at all.

9.3.2 Animal experiments

A number of animal experiments have been performed to address the role of the timing of operation and its effect on subsequent fertility. Pryor *et al.*[17] created undescended testes in rabbits a few days after birth. Orchidopexy was then performed at 21 days or 60 days, with histological analysis of the testis at 180 days. Both groups showed decreased tubular diameter and decreased number of germ cells per tubule. Since the normal testis descends at 9 days in the rabbit, both times for orchidopexy would allow potential secondary effects on the testis. The two orchidopexy groups gave similar results, suggesting that the interval between 21 and 60 days was not crucial for subsequent fertility. In addition, they were unable to identify any fall in paternity in adult males where the orchidopexy had been performed at 21 days.

Quinn[18] and colleagues[19] have used an elegant technique to study germ cell maturation after orchidopexy in rats. Since the spermatogonia contain only half the number of chromosomes compared with other cells, DNA flow cytometry can be used to estimate the number of mature (haploid) germ cells within the testis. Quinn cut the gubernaculum of neonatal rats to induce unilateral cryptorchidism, and then performed orchidopexy at 30 days (at the time of normal descent), 50 days ('pubertal') and 90 days (sexually mature). The percentage of haploid cells in the testis was compared with sham-operated controls at 120 days of age. The number of germ cells in adult rats was unaffected when orchidopexy was done at 30 days of age; diminished numbers of haploid cells could be reversed by orchidopexy at 50 days; but delay of orchidopexy to 90 days of age led to irreversible loss of germ cells. Quinn concluded that orchidopexy prior to adulthood reverses secondary degenerative changes in unilateral cryptorchidism.

Because orchidopexy in a pubertal rat could reverse or prevent germ cell loss, Quinn[18] speculated that orchidopexy in humans may not need to be done until puberty, because of the alleged risk of testicular atrophy mentioned earlier. We disagree with this interpretation, since his results equally could have produced the opposite conclusion: germ cell loss becomes manifest very shortly after normal descent of the testis (20–30 days in a rat), and is reversible initially and later irreversible. Therefore, one could argue that because human testis descends before birth (rather than at puberty), orchidopexy should be in early infancy. This divergence of opinions demonstrates not only the difficulty of extrapolation to humans from animal models, but also how completely different conclusions may be reached from the same evidence!

The role of the method of anchoring the testis has been studied by Bellinger *et al.*[20] Orchidopexy was performed in 35 adult rats using either absorbable (chromic catgut) suture, non-absorbable (nylon) suture or a classical dartos pouch technique without suture fixation. They found that the chromic catgut caused acute inflammation of the testis, leading to necrosis of some tubules and complete absence of spermatogenesis. Three 2/0 sutures were used, which would be a relatively large amount of irritating foreign material compared to the size of the rat testis. Nylon-fixed testes were adherent only at the suture and 29% had deficiency of spermatogenesis. Their dartos-pouch group were well fixed and spermatogenesis was normal in 96%. They concluded that suture fixation should be avoided because inflammatory reaction to the suture causes necrosis and germ cell damage. Their conclusion is important, although the inflammatory stimulus and risk of vascular damage would be much less in a larger human testis.

In a series of experiments, Juenemann *et al.*[21] and Kogan *et al.*[22,23] have studied the effect of cause and timing of cryptorchidism and the timing of orchidopexy on fertility. Initially they showed that neonatal surgical fixation of the testis within the abdomen produced a similar degree of infertility (as measured by paternity), as did cryptorchidism induced by postnatal treatment with 17-oestradiol.[21] Bilateral cryptorchidism (from either cause) suppressed fertility more than unilateral surgical maldescent, while unilateral orchidectomy did not inhibit fertility at all. They went on to show that the effect of oestradiol could be reversed partially with simultaneous treatment with hCG: the testes descended but subsequent fertility was still abnormal.[22] In a third study, Kogan *et al.*[23] surgically fixed the testes intra-abdominally at 11 days, and then compared the effects of orchidopexy at 21 with 28 days. After repair of the cryptorchid state at 21 days (the time of normal descent in a rat), the paternity rate was 72%, which was not significantly different from sham-operated controls (84%). This was in contrast to those rats having orchidopexy at 28 days, where subsequent paternity was significantly inhibited. Since the normal rat becomes sexually mature at 65 days, they postulated that this one week delay was roughly equivalent to several years of life in a child. They concluded, therefore, that early orchidopexy could be shown to improve fertility when performed early enough.

The conflicting human studies and animal experiments do not yet demonstrate clearly whether early surgery will preserve fertility in boys with undescended testis. The current view, that orchidopexy should be performed before secondary dysplasia develops, has evolved too recently to enable assessment of the long-term results of the policy. Such long-term clinical trials are still 10–20 years away from completion. Nevertheless, until definitive studies become available, it seems reasonable to assume that secondary degeneration may be a serious consequence of undescended testes which may be – at least partially – avoided by early surgery. The problem will be to separate secondary degeneration of the testis from primary testicular abnormalities as the cause of any subsequent decreased fertility.

9.3.3 Combined surgical and hormonal treatment

A promising new avenue of treatment which may improve fertility has been suggested by Hadziselimovic *et al.*[24] They treated 48 boys between 1.25 and 11 years of age with a long-acting analogue of LHRH (buserelin) on alternate days for 6 months. Their morphological and hormonal status was monitored closely. In the older boys a slightly increased level of serum testosterone was observed, but this was not seen in the younger boys. Orchidopexy was required in 83% of the boys because the hormone treatment failed to induce testicular descent. At orchidopexy, a biopsy was taken and these biopsies were compared with biopsies from normal children of similar ages. The number of germ cells per tubule was found to be significantly increased after buserelin treatment, such that in both bilateral and unilateral undescended testis the biopsies showed a normal number of germ cells in both groups. This is a significant observation which will require further research to confirm the findings. However, it does suggest that supplementary hormone treatment may turn out to be a useful adjunct to surgical placement of the testes in improving fertility potential.

9.3.4 Retractile testes

Few studies have addressed the subsequent fertility of boys with retractile testes. Rasmussen *et al.*[2] observed a cohort of 545 boys with undescended testes over a number of years. Ninety-one of these boys had bilateral undescended testes which were not operated upon, and which descended spontaneously into the scrotum after 10 years of age. When they were greater than 18 years of age, 45 of these young men were investigated for their fertility status. They had significantly decreased testicular volumes, and their sperm counts were below the lower limit of the normal range. The authors concluded that undescended testes that undergo spontaneous descent in adolescence have a significantly decreased potential for spermatogenesis, leading to relatively decreased fertility. In retrospect, it is not possible to know whether these boys had what might now be called 'retractile' or 'ascending' testes. However, since most surgeons believe that truly undescended testes would never descend into the scrotum it is quite likely that this group is intermediate between those with genuine undescended testis and normal males. These testes have been classified as either 'ascending' or 'retractile' testes by different authors making exact classification controversial. However, whatever their classification would be in current terminology they do show that spontaneous descent at puberty does not protect the child from subsequent decreased fertility in adult life. An important conclusion which could be reached from this study is that any testis which does not remain in the scrotum during childhood may suffer secondary degeneration regardless of its aetiology. This would be consistent with surgically-created cryptorchidism in animal studies where secondary degenerative changes occur which are very similar to that seen in the human.[18]

9.4 Malignancy

At present there are no figures which demonstrate whether early orchidopexy in children will reduce the risk of subsequent testicular tumours. No studies yet reported in the literature have a large enough group of children who have been operated on at a very young age. This is because the lag time between surgery and the likely onset of tumour is 30–40 years, which obviously is even greater than that for assessment of fertility.

Most studies present figures similar to those reported by Pike *et al.*[25] who found 9.5% of 724 men with a testicular tumour had a history of undescended testes (Table 9.2). Of the 69 men with a testicular tumour as well as a previous history of an undescended testis, 11 had never been operated upon. Orchidopexy during childhood or early adolescence had been

Table 9.2 Malignancy risk in men after orchidopexy

Authors	Patient numbers	Relative risk	UDT/cancer(%)
Gilbert and Hamilton[30]	over 7 000	48	11
Campbell[31]	1 413	64	11
Campbell[32]	12 535 824	35	11
Morrison[33]	596	8.8	–
Henderson *et al.*[34]	131	5.0	7.6
Schottenfeld *et al.*[35]	248	3.5	11.76
Pottern *et al.*[36]	271	3.7	9
Pike *et al.*[25]	724	–	9.5
Giwercman *et al.*[37]	506	4.7	–
Whitaker[38]	13 089	35	9.8
Strader *et al.*[39]	333	5.9	12
Benson *et al.*[40]	224	11.4	–

undertaken in 58. They found the age of orchidopexy was almost exactly equal to that expected in the total population undergoing orchidopexy, and therefore they could find no evidence that age provided a protective effect against the occurrence of tumours. However, they only had two patients who had surgery prior to 2 years of age and who developed a tumour, and more than half the patients had their orchidopexy after 10 years of age. Studies such as this demonstrate the difficulties in conducting epidemiological studies when there is such a long lag-time between the two events.

In a review of 34 men with testicular cancer and cryptorchidism, Jones *et al.*[26] found only nine had had prior orchidopexy, and seven of these had non-seminomas. By contrast, 16 out of 25 men with uncorrected maldescent had seminomas. Orchidopexy did not appear to have improved the prognosis or presentation because the non-seminomas were more advanced in staging. Mason *et al.*[27] recently studied 1191 men with primary germ cell tumours of the testis, seen at the Royal Marsden Hospital between 1977 and 1989. Inguinal or iliac node metastases were found in 22 men, seven of whom had had cryptorchidism and prior orchidopexy. The frequency of inguinal and iliac node involvement was significantly greater than expected in patients with a history of maldescent and orchidopexy, consistent with long-held surgical teaching that orchidopexy disrupts the normal lymphatic drainage of the testis. Nevertheless, previous surgery, apart from altering the management and follow-up of men with testicular cancer, does not seem to make the prognosis worse.

At present we must remain open-minded about whether early orchidopexy in infancy will decrease the risk for cancer formation. However, by locating the testes within the scrotum, subsequent diagnosis of a testicular tumour is made more straightforward. It is well recognized that an intrascrotal testis aids the early diagnosis of testicular tumours, and suggests that routine self-examination of the testis should be carried out in adolescence and young adult life.[28] Alternatively, adolescents with a past history of orchidopexy may be offered fine-needle biopsy for assessment of any premalignant degeneration, particularly carcinoma-*in-situ*, which is present in 2–3%.[29]

9.5 Conclusion

The current results of surgical treatment need to be considered carefully, taking into account the falling age of orchidopexy: the fertility and malignancy problems we see now are the result of orchidopexies done up to 40 years ago. It is presumed, but not yet proven, that operation in infancy will change this pattern dramatically: early evidence from testicular biopsies after orchidopexy supports this contention. Nevertheless, we will have to await the outcome of long-term studies to know for certain.

In general terms, we can define the features that affect the prognosis (cosmetic, fertility chance and malignancy risk)(Table 9.3). Good prognostic features include the position of the testis near the neck of the scrotum, ascending testes, retractile testes and (possibly) operation in early infancy. Bad features include primary dysplasia of the testis or epididymis, testes located in the abdomen or inguinal canal, an associated strangulated hernia (because of a higher risk of atrophy), and (possibly) operation delayed to late childhood or adolescence.

Table 9.3 Current prognostic features for undescended testes

Good prognosis	Bad prognosis
Testis near neck of scrotum	Primary testicular dysplasia
(?) Operation in early infancy	Testicular–epididymal separation
Ascending testes	Testis in abdomen/canal
Retractile testes	Strangulated hernia
	Operation in late childhood or adolescence

Greater understanding of the long-term implication for retractile and ascending testes must await prospective studies where these intermediate anomalies have been correctly classified and documented, something which is totally lacking in most reports to date.

References

1. Adamsen S, Bornesson B. Factors affecting the outcome of orchidopexy for undescended testis. *Acta Chir Scand* 1988; **154:** 529–33.

2. Rasmussen TB, Ingerslev HJ, Hostrup H. Natural history of the maldescended testis. *Horm Res* 1988; **30:** 164–6.
3. Werder EA, Illig R, Torresani T, *et al*. Gonadal function in young adults after surgical treatment of cryptorchidism. *Br Med J* 1976; **2:** 1357–9.
4. Wilson-Storey D, McGenity K, Dickson JAS. Orchidopexy: the younger the better? *J R Coll Surg (Edin)* 1990; **35:** 362–4.
5. Puri P, O'Donnell B. Semen analysis of patients who had orchidopexy at or after seven years of age. *Lancet* 1988; **ii:** 1051–2.
6. Thorup J, Kvist N, Larson P, *et al*. Clinical results of early and later operative correction of undescended testis. *Br J Urol* 1984; **56:** 322–5.
7. Gill B, Kogan S, Starr S, Reda E, Levitt S. Significance of epididymal and ductal anomalies associated with testicular maldescent. *J Urol* 1989; **142:** 556–8.
8. Marshall FF, Shermata DW. Epididymal abnormalities associated with undescended testes. *J Urol* 1979; **121:** 341.
9. Johansen TEB. Anatomy of the testis and epididymis in cryptorchidism. *Andrologia* 1987; **19:** 565–9.
10. Tamhne RC, Williams R. Orchidopexy at or after seven years of age. *Lancet* 1989; **i:** 49.
11. Atkinson PM, Epstein MT, Rippon AE. Plasma gonadotropins and androgens in surgically treated cryptorchid patients. *J Pediatr Surg* 1975; **10:** 27–33.
12. Cendron M, Keating MA, Huff DS, Koop CE, Snyder H McC, Duckett JW. Cryptorchidism, orchiopexy and infertility: a critical long-term retrospective analysis. *J Urol* 1989; **142:** 559–62.
13. Singh LP, Chaturvedi AK, Chawla F. A new approach in evaluation of fertility in surgically treated cryptorchids. *Acta Eur Fertil* 1987; **18:** 321–7.
14. Singer R, Dickerman Z, Sagiv M, Laron Z, Livni E. Endocrinological parameters and cell-mediated immunity postoperation for cryptorchidism. *Arch Androl* 1988; **20:** 153–7.
15. Kumar D, Bremner DN, Brown PW. Fertility after orchidopexy for cryptorchidism: a new approach to assessment. *Br J Urol* 1989; **64:** 516–20.
16. Chilvers C, Dudley NE, Gough MH, Jackson MB, Pike MC. Undescended testis: the effect of treatment on subsequent risk of subfertility and malignancy. *J Pediatr Surg* 1986; **21:** 691–6.
17. Pryor JL, Hurt GS, Caloras D, Turner TT, Flickinger CJ, Howards SS. Histologic analysis of orchidopexy in a cryptorchid rabbit model. *J Urol* 1988; **142:** 413–7.
18. Quinn FMJ; Evaluation of the scrotal testis before and after orchiopexy in experimental unilateral cryptorchidism. *J Pediatr Surg* 1991; **26:** 602–6.
19. Quinn FMJ, Crockard AD, Brown S. Reversal of degenerative changes in the scrotal testis after orchidopexy in experimental unilateral cryptorchidism. *J Pediatr Surg* 1991; **26:** 451–4.
20. Bellinger MF, Abromowitz H, Brantley S, Marshall G. Orchidopexy: an experimental study of the effect of surgical technique on testicular histology. *J Urol* 1989; **142:** 553–5.
21. Juenemann KP, Kogan BA, Abozeid MH. Fertility in cryptorchidism: an experimental model. *J Urol* 1986; **136:** 214–6.
22. Kogan BA, Gupta R, Juenemann KP. Fertility in cryptorchidism: further development of an experimental model. *J Urol* 1987; **137:** 128–31.
23. Kogan BA, Gupta R, Juenemann KP. Fertility in cryptorchidism: improved timing of fixation and treatment in an experimental model. *J Urol* 1987; **138:** 1046–7.
24. Hadziselimovic F, Huff D, Duckett J, *et al*. Long-term effect of luteinizing hormone-releasing hormone analogue (buserelin) on cryptorchid testes. *J Urol* 1987; **138:** 1043–5.

25. Pike MC, Chilvers C, Peckham MJ. Effect of age at orchidopexy on risk of testicular cancer. *Lancet* 1986; **i:** 1246–8.
26. Jones BKJ, Thornhill JA, O'Donnell B, *et al*. Influence of prior orchiopexy on stage and prognosis of testicular cancer. *Eur Urol* 1991; **19:** 201–3.
27. Mason MD, Featherstone T, Olliff J, Horwich A. Inguinal and iliac lymph node involvement in germ cell tumours of the testis: implications for radiological investigation and for therapy. *Clin Oncol (R Coll Radiol)* 1991; **3:** 147–50.
28. Palmer JM. The undescended testicle. *Endocrinol Metab Clin N Am* 1991: **20:** 231–40.
29. Giwercman A, Muller J, Skakkabaek NE. Cryptorchidism and testicular neoplasia. *Horm Res* 1988; **30:** 157–63.
30. Gilbert JB, Hamilton JB. Studies in malignant testis tumours. III Incidence and nature of tumours in ectopic testes. *Surg Gynecol Obstet* **71:** 731–43.
31. Campbell HE. Incidence of malignant growth of the undescended testicle: a critical and statistical study. *Arch Surg* 1942; **44:** 353–69.
32. Campbell HE. The incidence of malignant growth of the undescended testicle: A reply and reevaluation. *J Urol* 1959; **81:** 663–8.
33. Morrison AS. Cryptorchidism, hernia, and cancer of the testis. *J Natl Cancer Inst* 1976; **56:** 731–3.
34. Henderson BR, Benton B, Jing J, *et al*. Risk factors for cancer of the testis in young men. *Int J Cancer* 1979; **23:** 598–602.
35. Schottenfeld D, Warshauer ME, Sherlock S, *et al*. The epidemiology of testicular cancer in young adults. *Am J Epidemiol* 1980; **112:** 232–46.
36. Pottern LM, Brown LM, Hoover RN *et al*.Testicular cancer risk in boys with maldescended testis: A cohort study. *J Urol* 1985; **138:** 1214–6.
37. Giwercman A, Grindsted J, Hansen B, *et al*. Testicular cancer risk in boys with maldescended testis: A cohort study. *J Urol* 1987; **138:** 1214–6.
38. Whitaker RH. Neoplasia in cryptorchid men. *Sem Urol* 1988; **6:** 107–9.
39. Strader CK, Weiss NS, Daling JR, *et al*. Cryptorchidism, orchiopexy and the risk of testicular cancer. *Am J Epidemiol* 1988; **127:** 1013–18.
40. Benson RC, Beard CM, Kelalis PP, Kurland LT. Malignant potential of the cryptorchid testis. *Mayo Clin Proc* 1991; **66:** 372–8.

10

Conclusions and future developments

Testicular descent and undescended testes remain enigmas, although our understanding of both these processes has advanced considerably in the last 20 years.

A look at the evolution of testicular descent demonstrates that mammals have developed widely different anatomical solutions to the problem of storing cool spermatozoa. In particular, the site, form and physiology of the scrotum differ dramatically, yet most species show evidence of specific adaptations towards decreased gonadal and epididymal temperature. Our original aim in reviewing the evolutionary aspects was to see whether testicular descent could be divided into two separate phases, analogous to those seen in humans and laboratory animals. We hypothesized that, if the two steps were under different endocrine controls, this should be evident in their evolution because different mechanisms should evolve independently and probably separately in time. Not surprisingly, the evidence was a little too complex to confirm this suggestion outright, although there did appear to be a trend towards two separate steps.

Historical review of research done years ago proved to be a revelation, and the reader is urged to read these old papers directly, rather than rely on poor quality and inaccurate secondary sources. Hunter's description[1] is a landmark description of the gubernaculum that is still relevant today. The 'tails of Lockwood'[2] are never mentioned in Lockwood's original paper, but are thrust upon him by later writers.[3] Lockwood merely speculated that they may exist, without providing any direct evidence, in an attempt to account theoretically for the ectopic sites of gubernacular and testicular migration.

Perhaps the most revealing studies are the clear anatomical descriptions of the migration of the gubernaculum from the inguinal canal to the scrotum.[4] The importance of this migration phase has been forgotten and/or ignored in recent years, and had to be 'rediscovered', first by Backhouse[5] and then by Heyns.[6] Its key role in descent can be appreciated when one considers that the human gubernaculum is about 1 cm in diameter, yet the distance to the bottom of the scrotum is 4–5 cm.

With such a long distance to travel, we should be wondering why scrotal descent occurs at all, rather than why undescended testis is common (Figure 10.1).

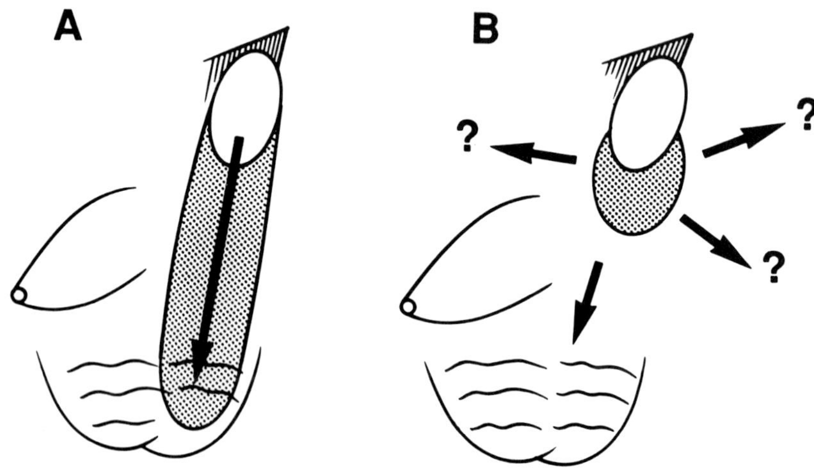

Figure 10.1 (A) Schema of how many clinicians view testicular descent, with the gubernaculum connecting the testis directly to the scrotum: descent seems a foregone conclusion and cryptorchidism a mystery. This incorrect view arose because the gubernaculum becomes secondarily attached to the scrotum after descent is complete. (B) The actual process of migration of a small gubernaculum across the groin is a precarious step which is not automatic: cryptorchidism seems, if not inevitable, at least not unexpected. Obviously there needs to be a mechanism to allow migration towards the scrotum; our postulate is that the genitofemoral nerve fulfils this role.

The first phase of testicular descent occurs between about 10–15 weeks of gestation and is linked to growth and enlargement of the gubernaculum, described by Wensing[7] as the swelling reaction. This growth of the gubernaculum anchors the testis close to the inguinal region during embryonic and fetal enlargement: in the female the lack of an enlarged gubernaculum allows the ovary to remain near the lumbar region during fetal growth. As the ovary recedes from the inguinal region, the gubernaculum becomes elongated and thin, later to become the ligament of the ovary and the round ligament. Although the ovary in the human ends up lying quite near the internal inguinal ring, the pathway of the round ligament reveals that in embryological terms the female gonad is distant from the inguinal canal. Unlike other animals that have a thin bicornuate uterus and perinephric ovaries, the human female has a short, solid uterus and pelvic ovaries: differences in the degree of müllerian duct fusion and uterine growth probably account for the lower position of the human ovary compared with many other mammals (Figure 10.2).

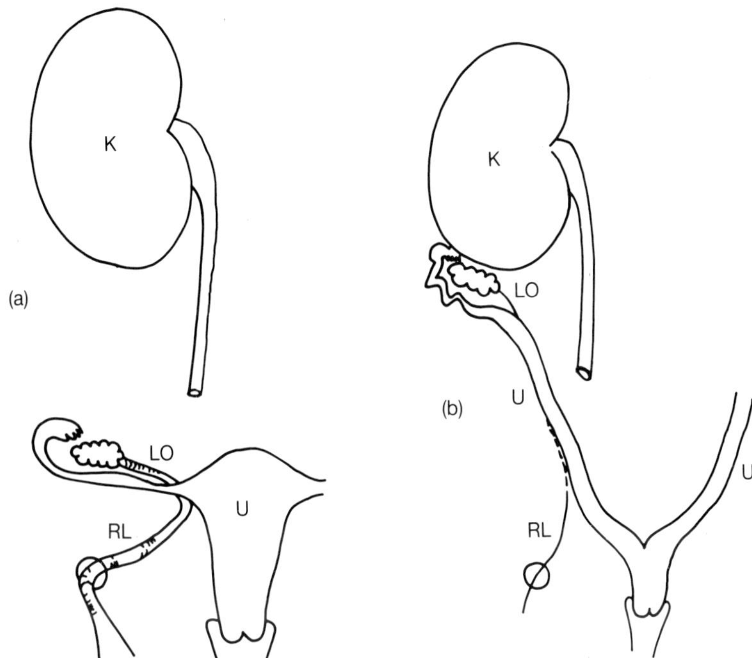

Figure 10.2 Diagram demonstrating the different position of the ovary in (A) humans, and (B) rodents, and its relation to the development of the uterus (U). Despite the proximity of the human ovary to the internal inguinal ring, the gubernacular ligaments are not foreshortened as in the male (K, kidney; LO, ligament of ovary; RL, round ligament). (Reproduced with permission from Reference 12.)

Transabdominal migration of the testis occurs at a different time and under different hormonal control than later inguino-scrotal descent. We have looked at a number of human and animal models, including the oestrogen-treated mouse, the androgen-insensitive mouse and human, and the human with persistent müllerian duct syndrome.

These models suggest not only that gubernacular swelling (and hence transabdominal descent) is independent of androgens, but also that it may be controlled by müllerian inhibiting substance. This is still a controversial view, as discussed in Chapter 2, and even the possibility that androgens might be important has been raised again recently.[8] By injecting pregnant rats with an anti-androgen (flutamide), they showed that testicular descent could be blocked. The anti-androgen was effective, however, only in the last week of gestation, during the phase of gubernacular growth. They postulated that androgens are important at this time, and implied this may indicate a role for testosterone in gubernacular enlargement. We would agree with their findings but interpret the data differently: since our proposal, described in Chapter 3, is that inguino-scrotal descent is controlled by androgens indirectly via the genitofemoral nerve, the androgens must first act on the nerve. Since known sexual dimorphisms in the spinal cord occur in the last week of gestation in rats,[9] this is the time we would predict that androgens would be important, as was found. In addition, although flutamide caused an 18–25% inhibition in gubernacular enlargement (measured by weight), 80% of the resultant undescended testes had traversed the abdomen and lodged ectopically in the groin. We suspect that gubernacular migration from the inguinal region may be controlled by a masculinized genitofemoral nerve, and therefore inhibition of normal 'masculinization' by flutamide would disrupt inguino-scrotal migration, as Spencer *et al.*[8] found.

The inguino-scrotal phase of descent, commencing between 26 and 28 weeks' gestation, appears to need androgenic stimulation as well as a normally 'masculinized' genitofemoral nerve. The precarious migration undertaken by the gubernaculum may be directed by the nerve, leading us to speculate that undescended testes may be caused by failure of the nerve to reach the scrotum, or rarely, by the nerve ending in an ectopic site (e.g. the perineum). The anatomy and physiology of the nerve will need extensive study in the future to determine its true role. It will be interesting to see whether the neurotransmitter we have identified in the nerve, calcitonin gene-related peptide (CGRP), can be shown to be a possible 'second messenger' for androgens acting on the gubernaculum. In addition, there is the future possibility that gubernacular migration may respond to exogenous CGRP, and lead to an entirely new way to induce testicular descent nonsurgically (Figure 10.3).

In discussing the classification of undescended testes, it is the testis in the superficial inguinal pouch that is the most difficult to understand. By comparison, it is straightforward to imagine that testes arrested in the line of descent have a possible primary deficiency of androgens and ectopic testes have migrated to the wrong place (secondary to a misplaced genitofemoral nerve?). The superficial inguinal pouch does not appear to be 'ectopic' and yet it is off the line of descent. At surgery, the gubernaculum in these cases usually is attached just outside the neck of the scrotum, perhaps secondary to failure of the genitofemoral nerve to reach the scrotum. The lateral displacement of the testis and processus vaginalis may well be a passive result of physical pressure, or alternatively may be forced upon the testis because of a fascial barrier preventing its entry into the scrotum. Further research is needed to resolve these possibilities.

The 'retractile' testis is another dilemma, creating a major controversy over whether it is normal or abnormal. The criteria devised by Wyllie[10] (see page 104), imply that some retractile testes are abnormal, while others never need treatment. This apparent heterogeneity complicates clinical decision-making enormously. The cause of retractile testes is unknown, but their response to hormone (LHRH or hCG) treatment

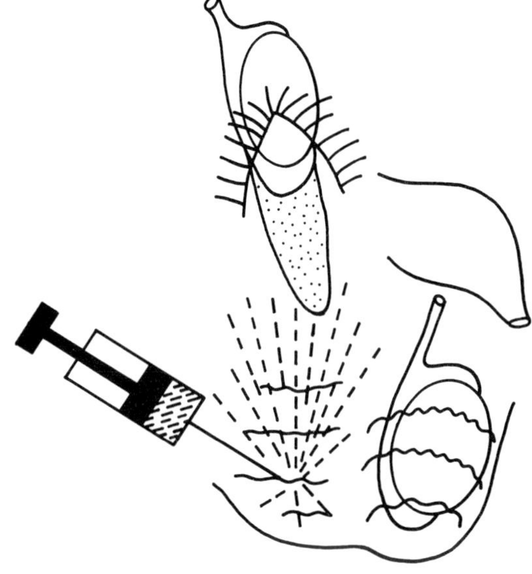

Figure 10.3 A speculative schema showing that the CGRP might be used as a 'hormone' treatment for undescended testes. If further research confirmed our suggestion that CGRP controls gubernacular migration, exogenous CGRP might be used to induce gubernacular migration (and hence testicular descent) artificially.

suggests a partial deficiency of androgens. Much fruitful knowledge about this common clinical problem should come out of longitudinal follow-up studies, as currently being done at the John Radcliffe Hospital in Oxford.

As if retractile testes were not difficult enough, we are faced now with an apparently new enigmatic subgroup of cryptorchidism, known as 'ascending' testes. This intriguing phenomenon occurs in boys with postnatal descent of the testes, usually in the first 12 weeks after birth. With subsequent growth of the boy, the spermatic cord fails to elongate in proportion to body size, giving the impression that the testis is rising back out of the scrotum.

At present, we remain ignorant of the cause, natural history and consequences of 'ascending' testes, let alone the need for treatment. A major new goal for the future is to categorize this variant precisely so that rational decisions can be made about whether treatment is required.

The frequency of cryptorchidism probably is rising, although the epidemiological explanation for this is obscure. Likewise, the causes of undescended testis remain largely unknown, except for a few rare situations, where recent research has revealed some putative explanations: in prune belly syndrome and posterior urethral valves, bladder enlargement is likely to disrupt the entry of the testis into the internal inguinal ring; in exomphalos and gastroschisis, the abdominal pressure may be lower than normal either acutely (with rupture) or chronically; spina bifida may lead to derangement of the genitofemoral nerve, and hence interfere with gubernacular migration; while in cerebral palsy, maldescent is likely to be secondary to an upper motor neurone lesion affecting the cremaster muscle, leading to pathologically 'retracted' testes.

For the otherwise normal boy with an undescended testis, the cause is probably local mechanical factors. We speculate that minor derangement of one genitofemoral nerve may cause the testis to remain in the groin, while true ectopic testes are likely to be secondary to an aberrant peripheral pathway of the genitofemoral axons. A few undescended testes result from primary gonadal (and hence hormonal) deficiency.

The effects of cryptorchidism are secondary to the abnormally high temperature experienced by the non-scrotal testis, which leads initially to physiological abnormalities (such as deficiency of postnatal secretion of testosterone and MIS), and later to morphological derangement. Macroscopic dysplasia with loss of germ cells and a 5–10 fold increase in the cancer risk is the ultimate consequence, and these latter problems remain the primary reasons for offering treatment.

With the recent observations that germ cells are depleted during infancy, the recommended age for surgery has fallen stepwise to this age, with the hope that infertility and testicular cancer will be avoided in young adult life. These high hopes and ideals need to be kept in perspective, however, since that is all they are. The central dilemma facing clinicians dealing with cryptorchid infants is that there is no definite proof that the treatment will work. Despite many attempts to find out sooner or by alternative means, we are caught at present in a lag-phase between the initiation (on a large scale) of infantile surgery and its long-term results in grown men. Nevertheless, the limited evidence available is full of hope that repair in infancy will improve the prognosis for the adult testis.

We describe our own methods of clinical examination in detail in Chapter 6. The two most important points worth remembering about the physical examination, apart from it being difficult, are that to find an inguinal testis, the surgeon needs to know the bony landmarks (to identify the inguinal canal and superficial inguinal pouch), and that the testis is mobile. Many a time have students proudly announced in the outpatient clinic that they have located an inguinal testis, only to be crestfallen when they realize that they have found an enlarged inguinal lymph node. Surprisingly, many people do not know that the undescended testis is extremely mobile within its undescended processus vaginalis, making it hard to find unless one looks deliberately for something mobile. We give some useful criteria for distinguishing truly undescended from retractile testes, although even with simple criteria, the assessment can be difficult.

There is not yet concensus on what a retractile testis is, or how to decide whether any individual testis is retractile, undescended or normal.

Investigation of impalpable testes is an interesting and controversial area, with many new techniques (e.g. laparoscopy), competing with each other and with surgical exploration as the optimal method. With the rapid advance of interventional laparoscopy, diagnostic laparoscopy should also advance with new instruments. The exact role of each of these methods is uncertain because many are new and untried, and the technology is developing so quickly it is hard to guess what will be next.

The surgical technique of orchidopexy has not changed much in the last decade, since the introduction of subcuticular, dissolvable sutures. Exotic methods of external fixation of the testis have been abandoned long ago in favour of simple internal fixation: either 'button-holing' the testis through the scrotal fascia or light anchoring to the midline septal tissues. Rapid changes have occurred in the child's experience of surgery, with day-case procedures, no painful premedication injection and local (cream) anaesthesia for induction of anaesthetic (to avoid 'the needle'), and regional analgesia for the operative site afterwards. Waterproof and effectively adherent dressings allow immediate bathing and avoid external wound contamination, which now is a more serious risk because the patients are still in nappies.

The various procedures available for the intra-abdominal testis are described, although the best choice is not yet clear: most surgeons are still using the operation they know best, rather than the latest technique. Micro-surgical transfer has not yet replaced older and more conservative approaches, perhaps because intra-abdominal testes are not common enough to allow surgeons to develop the special facility required. Two-stage procedures remain popular, with the two-stage 'Fowler–Stephens' operation receiving much current attention.

Hormone treatment has waned in popularity in recent years with numerous clinical trials demonstrating poor efficacy except for retractile testes. It is a great irony, and a measure of the craving for better alternatives to surgery, that hormone therapy was pushed so hard for nearly 60 years, despite being based on a model of precocious puberty. Most reviews of hormone treatment cite Engle[11] as a landmark in the English literature, for showing that immature macaque testes could be induced to descend with crude pituitary hormone extracts. Few advocates realized that the macaque testis descends prenatally, then reascends after birth to the groin until puberty. Hormonal treatment merely induced secondary pubertal descent, analogous to that currently seen in retractile testes.

The main roles for hormonal therapy in the future may be as a diagnostic test for retractile testes in older boys, or as an adjunct to surgery to stimulate germ cell maturation.

The long-term outlook for a cryptorchid infant, treated well, should be a significant improvement in fertility and reduction of cancer risk later in life. We will, however, be waiting for a few years yet before there are large clinical studies to support this optimistic view. The possibility of alternative therapies arising from the research described in Chapters 2 and 3 remains uncertain: new understanding, however, should help us resolve the many unanswered questions about this fascinating clinical problem.

References

1. Hunter J. A description of the situation of the testis in the foetus, with its descent into the scrotum. In: *Observations on Certain Parts of the Animal Oeconomy*. London, 1786: pp. 1–26.
2. Lockwood CB. Development and transition of the testis, normal and abnormal. *J Anat Physiol* 1888; **22:** 505–41.
3. McGregor AL. The third inguinal ring. *Surg Gynecol Obstet* 1929; **49:** 273–307.
4. Cleland J. *The Mechanism of the Gubernaculum Testis*. Prize thesis. Edinburgh: MacLachlan & Stewart, 1856.
5. Backhouse KM. Embryology of testicular descent and maldescent. *Urol Clin N Am* 1982; **9:** 315–25.
6. Heyns CF. The gubernaculum during testicular descent in the human fetus. *J Anat* 1987; **153:** 93–112.
7. Wensing CJG. Testicular descent in some domestic mammals. III. Search for the factors that regulate the gubernacular reaction. *Proc Kon Ned Akad Wetensch C* 1973; **76:** 196–202.
8. Spencer JR, Torrado T, Sanchez RS, Vaughan ED, Imperato-McGinley J. Effects of flutamide and finasteride on rat testicular descent. *Endocrinology* 1991; **129:** 741–8.
9. Breedlove SM. Hormonal control of the anatomical specificity of motoneuron-to-muscle innervation in rats. *Science* 1989; **227:** 1357–9.
10. Wyllie GG. The retractile testis. *Med J Aust* 1984; **140:** 403–5.
11. Engle ET. Experimentally induced descent of the testis in the Macacus monkey by hormones from the anterior pituitary and pregnancy urine. *Endocrinology* 1932; **16:** 513–20.
12. Hutson JM, Williams MPL, Fallat ME, Attah A. Testicular descent: new insights into its hormonal control. In: *Oxford Reviews of Reproductive Biology*, 12 (Milligan SR, ed). Oxford, Oxford University Press, 1990: pp 1–56.

Index